THE
COLLAGEN
Diet

Rejuvenate Skin, Strengthen Joints and Feel Younger by Boosting Collagen Intake and Production

Pamela Schoenfeld, MS, RD, LDN

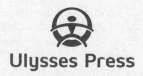

Ulysses Press

Published in the United States by:
Ulysses Press
P.O. Box 3440
Berkeley, CA 94703
www.ulyssespress.com

ISBN: 978-1-61243-832-0
Library of Congress Control Number: 2018944082

Printed in Canada by Marquis Book Printing
10 9 8 7 6 5 4 3 2 1

Acquisitions: Casie Vogel
Managing editor: Claire Chun
Editors: Shayna Keyles, Lauren Harrison
Proofreader: Renee Rutledge
Index: Sayre Van Young
Front cover design: Ashley Prine
Honeycomb artwork: © Lesik Vitaliy/shutterstock.com
Production: Jake Flaherty

Distributed by Publishers Group West

Contents

PART 1: WHY CARE ABOUT COLLAGEN? 1

Introduction. 2

CHAPTER 1
Collagen, the Building Material of Life. 9

CHAPTER 2
Historical Use of Collagen 16

CHAPTER 3
Why Is Collagen Protein Needed in the
Modern-Day Diet? 22

CHAPTER 4
Beauty from Within 33

CHAPTER 5
Keep Moving with Collagen. 57

CHAPTER 6
Collagen and Your Gut Reaction 72

CHAPTER 7
Could Collagen Each Day Help Keep the
Cardiologist Away?. 78

CHAPTER 8
Weighing In on Collagen...........................83

CHAPTER 9
Collagen: The Right Protein for Optimizing
Blood Sugar 92

CHAPTER 10
Amino Acids and Collagen........................102

CHAPTER 11
Collagen at Every Age, Every Stage................114

CHAPTER 12
How Much Collagen Protein Is Right for You?.........124

CHAPTER 13
Collagen Supplements: Frequently Asked Questions 130

CHAPTER 14
Collagen's Supporting Cast 140

PART 2: RECIPES.........................149

CHAPTER 15
Collagen: Easy and Delicious Ways to Get More 150

BREAKFAST.................................... 153
Omelet with Sweet Potato Twirls 153
Berry Oatmeal Bake 155
Pumpkin Protein Pancakes 156
Honey-Banana Protein Pancakes 158
Blueberry Protein Pancakes....................... 160
Coconut Collagen Coffee "Creamer"................. 161

APPETIZERS 163
Guacamole. 163
Bloody Mary Aspic with Shrimp 164
Shrimp Cocktail Mold 166
"Refried" Black Bean Dip 167

SOUPS 169
Poultry Bone Broth 169
Beef Bone Broth 171
Easy Chicken Soup 173
Italian Wedding Soup 175
Cream of Vegetable Soup 177

SIDES AND SALADS 179
Salmon Skin Salad 179
Lemon Tahini Salad Dressing and Dip 181
Lentil-Parsley Salad 182
Mashed Potatoes 184
Roasted Vegetables 185

MAIN DISHES 186
Ginger Chicken Curry 186
Sesame-Glazed Chicken Wings 188
Beef Stew 190
Italian Meatballs 192
Creole Cod 195
Simple Pan-Seared Salmon 197
Baked Falafel 199
Coconut Chickpea Curry 201

SNACKS AND DESSERTS 203
Pumpkin Seed Chocolate Collagen Protein Bars 203
Coconut Chocolate Chia "Pudding" 205
Paleo Chocolate-Avocado Freezer Fudge 207
Coconut Collagen "Cookies" 208
Protein-Powered Coconut-Pecan "Fudge" 210
Herbal Tea or Fruit Juice Gummies 211
Paleo Candy Sour Gummies 212

SMOOTHIES. 214
Whey-Collagen Protein Smoothie 214
Coconut Pineapple Smoothie 216
Blueberry Collagen Smoothie 217
Green Smoothie. 218
Strawberry Collagen Smoothie 219

Conclusion 220

Conversion Charts 222

Selected References 223

Index 227

Acknowledgments 234

About the Author 234

PART 1

WHY CARE ABOUT COLLAGEN?

Introduction

Boneless, skinless chicken breasts, skinless fish fillets, and lean meats have been the "healthy choices" of diet-conscious individuals for more than three decades. Most of my clients in my nutrition practice tell me that they eat only skinless poultry, even removing the skin from a store-bought rotisserie chicken, anticipating that I will almost certainly commend them for their healthy choice.

When I tell them that the skin they're tossing in the garbage (or giving to their dog) actually contains a valuable nutrient that is difficult to obtain from other foods, a puzzled look comes over their faces. They ask, doesn't removing the skin do away with unwanted fat and calories? While this can be the case, the skin of the chicken contains an abundance of collagen protein that can support the health of their own skin, bones, and joints. And chicken fillets, like all skinless meats, only contain a very small amount of collagen protein.

Often, clients admit that they find it difficult to eat chicken skin because *they simply don't like it.* I agree that it is difficult at first to enjoy eating something that you've almost never eaten before—even the popular fried chicken nuggets targeted at children have always been stripped of the skin. I persistently suggest they might want to try roasting some tasty marinated chicken wings or making a delicious homemade soup with the leftovers from a rotisserie chicken. And once I educate them on the many ways their bodies can benefit from the collagen protein supplied by the parts of the chicken they previously discarded, they're eager to learn additional ways to get collagen in their diets.

Why do I encourage my clients to eat the chicken skin along with the meat? Many informed nutritionists now understand that there are benefits to eating the skin that covers the breast, wings, legs, and thighs, together with all of the other parts of the chicken. My personal practice is to first enjoy the crispy skin of a freshly roasted chicken (after discarding the majority of fat that drips into the pan), followed by eating a leg and thigh. What better way to have a delicious meal and get the health benefits from the collagen protein found almost exclusively in the skin, bones, and connective tissues of the chicken, and for that matter, any other animal?

Why should you be concerned about getting plenty of collagen in your diet? The simplest answer is that our bodies contain a lot of it! Collagen is a structural protein that makes up almost one-third of our tissues, making it a major player in the human body—essential for our joints, cartilage, and tendons; our bones, skin, hair, nails, and teeth; and even our blood vessels and eyes. All of these tissues contain one or more types of collagen. Collagen synthesis, or the formation of new collagen, is absolutely required by all of these vital tissues, especially during growth and the repair and recovery periods following injury or disease.

Perhaps more importantly, collagen gives these tissues the elasticity, flexibility, and strength needed to prevent degeneration in the first place. With less breakdown and more regeneration, skin stays more youthful, hair resists breakage, bones are more resilient, joints better resist wear and tear, and nails grow longer and stronger. Often called the "glue" that holds the body together, adequate, high-quality collagen keeps us from becoming floppy, leaky, and creaky! Consuming collagen is an important way to support the integrity of the collagen that the body manufactures.

Consuming collagen protein also increases the supply of amino acids, or protein building blocks, that our bodies need to deal with environmental toxins and synthesize critical antioxidants. Additionally, exciting new research demonstrates collagen protein may help with weight management, sleep problems, diabetes, high blood pressure, inflammation, and even digestive issues. And dietary collagen protein appears to enhance muscle growth, reduce pain and inflammation, and support joint integrity, which is good news whether you are a competitive or even a weekend athlete. It truly is a remarkably versatile substance that can improve many common health conditions and elevate overall wellness and vitality.

Because our bodies can synthesize collagen using the amino acids found in other proteins that we eat, consuming collagen protein is technically optional. Yet consuming dietary collagen offers a myriad of health benefits in part because it stimulates the body to make more of its own collagen, forestalling wrinkles, arthritis, muscle and bone loss, and general bodily wear and tear.

My Own Collagen Protein Experience

When you think of collagen protein, what first comes to your mind? Perhaps, as I once did, you initially think of stronger nails and more youthful skin. That's just the beginning. My own understanding of collagen protein and what it can do has evolved substantially over the past few decades, along with the leading research that is uncovering more and more benefits of including collagen protein in our diet.

As a teenager, I bought into the Knox Unflavored Gelatin advertisements in the 1970s that promised stronger, longer fingernails by consuming just one packet of their gelatin drink mix per day. Gelatin is made from the skin and bones of animals and is almost pure collagen protein. It is also a main ingredient in products like Jell-O. My fingernails had always been prone to splitting and breaking, and the various nail treatments I brushed on never seemed to help. Knox Gelatin seemed like the answer to getting those long, strong nails I envied in my high school girlfriends. So I conducted my own dietary experiment by consuming Knox, hoping to see quick and measurable results. Unfortunately, not finding much of a difference after a few weeks, I prematurely dismissed it as a beauty fad and resigned myself to having slow-growing, weak nails. (Plus, those individual packages of gelatin were somewhat pricey for my hard-earned money!) Yet had I patiently stuck with this beauty habit long-term, I probably would have seen results, as I do now. I'll discuss how gelatin can improve nails in Chapter 4.

During my first-semester college anatomy and physiology course, I became fascinated by the science behind how the nutrients we eat impact the biochemical workings of our bodies—so fascinated that I promptly changed my major from pre-med to nutrition research. I remember reading in my introductory nutrition textbook that the protein in collagen was "incomplete" and by definition lacked one or more of the nine essential amino acids. Collagen is missing the essential amino acid tryptophan and contains low amounts of iso-leucine, threonine, and methionine. Therefore, collagen cannot by itself satisfy the protein requirements of the human body. Aha, I concluded, that is why my nail experiment failed: Gelatin is a type of collagen and an incomplete protein, so it offers no nutritional value on its own. This proved to be wrongful thinking!

In my early thirties, I began to look into facial creams to ward off the signs of aging. Looking and feeling young became important to me, especially since I had been a sun-lover in my teens and twenties, and was, at this time, a mother of three operating on a sleep deficit. Products that touted collagen as an active ingredient grabbed my attention. Knowing that skin is largely made of collagen protein, I thought applying it topically would offer a way to nourish and replenish it. I tried a few of these products, hoping they would prove effective.

Not long after these collagen-containing creams and lotions became popular, articles began appearing in women's magazines stating there was zero benefit to applying collagen to the skin. The fact is that collagen is a very large molecule, making it impossible for the skin to assimilate and utilize it from the outside. These creams were at best just over-priced moisturizers, and according to dermatologists at the time, plain old petroleum jelly performed equally well. Skin care has advanced by leaps and bounds since the 1980s, offering a myriad of topical choices that contain active ingredients, such as collagen peptides (collagen that has been broken into smaller pieces), which can penetrate the skin. And while many of these products do offer anti-aging benefits, it is becoming clearer that health and beauty truly begins from within.

Fast-forward to today. Having completed my master's degree in nutrition and practiced for a decade as a registered dietitian nutritionist, I know that a lot of what I learned in the late 1970s about nutrition has not stood up to scientific scrutiny. For example, it was wrong to dismiss collagen's important role in human nutrition. The fact is, collagen protein is proving to be one of the most valuable contributors to a well-balanced diet!

It is true that collagen protein does not contain the full complement of amino acids needed to make many of the structural proteins in the body, and that by itself, collagen cannot support the growth and repair of our bodies. Yet collagen protein offers amazing benefits when included in a well-balanced diet. These benefits can start even before we are born and continue throughout our entire lives.

What You'll Learn in This Book

If you're like many of my clients, you may find the vast array of nutritional supplements overwhelming. Every week, another new supplement comes on the market with promises that it can reduce the risk for one or more diseases, slow aging, or give you a slimmer and more youthful body. These claims may have a basis in truth but are often hugely overstated. To add to the confusion, even top nutritionists and doctors disagree on whether nutritional supplements are beneficial, simply a waste of money, or potentially dangerous to your health. You want to make sure what you are putting into your body is safe, will give you the results you expect, and is backed by legitimate clinical research and experience.

As a registered dietitian nutritionist, I have studied and observed firsthand the benefits of foods and nutritional supplements on human health for over two decades. I can confidently endorse collagen protein as a proven winner. It's not just hype; collagen protein is the real deal.

And like my clients, I want you to really understand what collagen protein can do for you, which foods naturally contain it, and how you can easily include more of it in your diet using uncomplicated yet delicious recipes that contain other healthful ingredients. I've provided a number of recipes in Part 2 to make it a snap to get your daily dose of collagen protein.

In Chapter 1, you'll get an overview of what an amazingly versatile protein collagen is and how our bodies depend on it. In Chapter 2, we'll cover a brief history of how humans have valued and used collagen protein for thousands of years. Chapter 3 will examine why we need collagen protein in our diet. Chapters 4 through 7 will discuss the many ways collagen can support health, beauty, and performance—from our skin, bones, joints, and muscles to our cardiovascular and digestive systems. In Chapters 8 and 9, you'll learn how dietary collagen can be helpful if you have weight or blood sugar concerns. Chapter 10 is about those important little amino acids—glycine, proline, and arginine—and why collagen protein can aid in detoxification and even mental health. In Chapter 11, you'll learn the benefits of collagen protein across the lifespan. I cover how to decide how much collagen to consume daily, which foods naturally contain it, and how the vast array of supplements containing collagen protein differ in Chapters 12 and 13. And since collagen protein does not operate alone, I'll discuss the other nutrients that are beneficial for your own healthy collagen production in Chapter 14.

Collagen protein is truly a superfood that everyone at every age can benefit from—you won't have to miss a day without it!

CHAPTER 1

Collagen, the Building Material of Life

Collagen is an amazingly versatile protein. It is the single most abundant protein in the human body, making up over 30 percent. The major constituent of our connective tissues, collagen gives our bodies their strength and provides the structural integrity for our tissues and organs. It is a unique protein in many ways: For one, it is rich in glycine, proline, and hydroxyproline, three amino acids that are relatively uncommon in other proteins in our bodies. (Hydroxyproline is actually unique to collagen.) Amino acids are the basic building blocks that combine to form all of the human body's proteins, and they're typically designated as either essential or nonessential. Essential amino acids must be supplied by what we eat and drink, whereas nonessential amino acids can be made by our bodies, even if we do not get them from our diets.

While glycine and proline are not included in the group of nine essential amino acids, evidence is accumulating that these two "nonessential" amino acids perform several beneficial roles in the human body. Importantly, they are considered two of nine "*conditionally* essential" amino acids. A conditionally essential amino acid may not be required in the diet for someone in good health. However, a conditionally essential amino acid often becomes essential during periods of illness or stress. Stress basically means that the body is facing a challenge that puts it out of homeostasis, a state of balance, resulting in the body working overtime to try to restore its balance. Maybe you're like me and you don't always feel in balance—you get too little sleep, eat on the run, underdo or overdo the exercise, or maybe you're just getting older. These are things that can put your body under stress. Telltale signs that your body is working to restore balance include fatigue, pain, sleep problems, mood changes, and even weight gain.

Types of Collagen

Twenty-eight different types of collagen have been identified in the human body, but about 90 percent of our collagen is one of four types: I, II, III, and IV. These differ in their biological function and in which genes code for them, but the three predominant collagen types, I, II, and III, share a common molecular structure: the triple-stranded helix. Picture this helix as a braided rope, made from three strands of amino acid "chains" coiled around each other and connected by loose bonds. This braided-rope configuration gives collagen its unique ability to be flexible yet exceedingly strong. The "rope" can consist of three identical, two identical and one different, or three different amino acid chains, determining the type of collagen.

The most abundant type of collagen in our bodies is type I, the sole type of collagen in tendons and bones, which contain 80 percent and 30 percent collagen, respectively. Tendons attach a muscle either to a bone or to another muscle, and tendons need to withstand enormous stretching without breaking. Type I collagen is perfectly designed for that purpose—ounce for ounce, it is stronger than steel! Type I is also the predominant type of collagen in the skin (75 percent collagen), and largely makes up the layers of skin cells that lie just beneath what is visible on the surface. The visible skin is largely keratin, a protein with a different amino sequence from collagen. Type I collagen is also found in the cornea of the eye, the dentin of the teeth, and most connective tissues.

Tissues containing type I collagen are clearly quite different from each other—some are elastic and flexible, while others are stiff and strong. Collagen is an incredibly versatile building material and its mechanical properties are largely determined by the modification of its structure, even while retaining the same basic chemical composition. For example, in bone and dentin, the stiffness of collagen is further increased through the incorporation of minerals, including calcium and magnesium.

Type II collagen is found exclusively in the cartilage layered across the surfaces of the joints, allowing our bones to "glide" against each other. It is also found in the windpipe, voice box, and air passages in the lungs, allowing them to hold their shape but remain pliable. Additionally, it is found in a few other places, including the cornea of the eyes and in the ears.

Type III collagen is found everywhere type I is, with the exception of the bones, tendons, and a few specialized tissues, such as the cornea. Type III, and type I to a lesser extent, form the main structural components of the blood vessels (which are 40 percent collagen). When we begin life, our skin consists of a high percentage of type III collagen, about 50 percent, and the remainder is mainly type I. By adulthood, only 10 to 20 percent of the collagen present in skin is type III. The intestines, like the blood vessels, contain slightly more of type III as compared with type I. The uterine wall also contains type III.

Type IV collagen differs from types I, II, and III in that it does not form the same triple-stranded helix structure. Instead, it is laid down in a delicate web-like pattern to form the major component of the "basement membrane." The basement membrane is essentially a layer of tissue that defines the boundaries of the skin, muscles, and fat, and it serves as functional tissue in organs, including the kidneys and the digestive tract.

The amino acid chains that make up collagen types I, II, and III are further connected through a process called "cross-linking" that reinforces the molecular structure of the collagen proteins—essentially, this makes the collagen more rigid and less flexible. Cross-linking of our collagen increases as we age, causing the proteins to become stronger and less pliable over time. Excessive cross-linking can lead to an abnormal rigidity that often leads to clouding of the cornea, hardening of the arteries, and reduced mobility and flexibility in muscles and joints. While this process is associated with aging, the rate at which it happens is somewhat under our control. Medical researchers have shown that excessive sun exposure, cigarette smoking, and elevated blood sugar, things you already know should be avoided, all cause an undesirable acceleration in cross-linking.

How Collagen Forms in the Body

Formation of collagen, also called collagen synthesis, proceeds quite differently from the synthesis of other proteins in our bodies. It starts with the creation of precursor proteins called "procollagens." Of the 20 different amino acids that make up procollagen proteins, three— glycine, proline, and lysine—are considered the most important, both for procollagen construction and ultimately the unique characteristics of collagen. The synthesis of procollagens takes place inside one of three cell types: in the fibroblasts (cells that make connective tissue), the osteoblasts (cells that make bone), or the chondroblasts (cells that further develop into cartilage cells).

After winding together in groups of three to form a characteristic triple helix, the procollagen is sent outside of the cell to be modified into mature collagen. In this extracellular space, hydroxyl groups combine with much of the proline and lysine, a process called hydroxylation, generating the bonds that stabilize the functional collagen protein. Glycine accounts for one of every three amino acids, and its small size allows the longer amino acids to fit nicely within the inner part of the final collagen molecule.

It is vitally important that our bodies are able to produce ample amounts of good-quality collagen. Good-quality collagen underlies the strength and structure of our bodies; the integrity of our skin, hair, and nails, which are the physical barriers against outside threats, including harsh weather and microorganisms; and the basic functioning of all of our organs and blood vessels. Good nutrition is the foundation for producing good-quality collagen, and while consuming diverse sources of protein is necessary, it is not sufficient. Vitamins, minerals, and essential fats are equally important.

Zinc and vitamin A are needed by the cells that create and then secrete procollagen. During procollagen formation, vitamin C and iron are required for the hydroxylation of proline and lysine. Copper is needed to form the bonds between the lysine molecules that crosslink and further stabilize the collagen molecule. Zinc is required by enzymes that degrade and remodel collagen, a normal process that is especially important during wound healing. Manganese is needed for the activation of an enzyme that the body requires to make proline. Despite the abundance of food in this country, it is not uncommon for individuals to be low in one or more of these nutrients, with consequences for healthy collagen production.

When Collagen Production Is Interrupted

To gain a better understanding of what happens when the body's normal production of collagen is interrupted, we'll briefly look at what are called collagen or connective tissue diseases.

Relatively uncommon today, scurvy is a connective tissue disease caused by a dietary deficiency of vitamin C. Because collagen synthesis requires vitamin C, a diet devoid of fresh fruits and vegetables can result in this very serious but usually reversible condition. Symptoms begin with bleeding gums and poor wound healing, and can progress to hemorrhaging and eventually death if not detected early enough. Because vitamin C is destroyed as foods are heated, fresh or lightly cooked fruits and vegetables are an essential part of every balanced diet.

A somewhat different connective tissue disease is Ehlers-Danlos syndrome, occurring in about one in five thousand people. This genetic condition is due to a defect in collagen and connective tissue synthesis and structure. People afflicted with Ehlers-Danlos syndrome often develop hypermobile joints, fragile skin that stretches easily, and an increased propensity for bruising, although the clinical picture is quite diverse.

Certain autoimmune conditions are thought to be caused by the immune system attacking the fibroblasts, one of the three types of cells that produce collagen. Rheumatoid arthritis, which causes painful swollen joints, and scleroderma, which leads to tight skin and a limited range of motion in the joints, are connective tissue diseases in this category.

Finally, even the normal process of aging is marked by a 1 percent reduction in collagen synthesis each year, decreasing the skin's ability to repair itself and causing the skin to become thinner and more fragile. Wrinkling, while inevitable the longer we live, is accelerated when the cross-linking of collagen proceeds beyond what is normal. Increased cross-linking also contributes to the stiff joints many of us experience by the time we're in our sixties.

The good news is that the ravages of time can be interrupted and possibly even reversed by adopting healthful practices, including sensible sun exposure, moderate exercise, restorative sleep, and optimal nutrition—and yes, a diet rich in collagen. Time marches on, but being proactive will allow you to stay younger and more active. I just turned 60 myself, but I feel like I did when I was in my forties. People often don't believe my age until I show them the photos of my darling grandson!

One thing I have seen firsthand is that it is never too late to start an age-defying diet and lifestyle. That's why I wrote this book—so you, too, can increase the life in your years!

CHAPTER 2

Historical Use of Collagen

If you're now excited and ready to learn exactly what collagen protein can do for you, you may want to skip to Chapter 4. While the information in these next two chapters is quite fascinating, the remainder of the book more specifically discusses the health benefits of collagen protein. If you do skip ahead, you will definitely want to come back to these two short chapters to learn even more reasons to love collagen protein!

Through all of recorded history, humans have valued collagen protein for a variety of purposes. The word collagen comes from the Greek word *kolla*, meaning "glue." And while the first documented uses of collagen were as adhesives in the manufacturing of goods, it soon became highly valued for its medicinal and health-promoting properties.

Traditionally, humans have derived collagen from the long, slow boiling of the skin, hide, scales, bones, joints, and cartilaginous and connective tissues of land and sea animals. Before boiling, these tissues would typically be treated with an acid or basic solution to facilitate the release of greater quantities of collagen protein. Medicinally, collagen protein was first utilized in the form of gelatin, produced by simmering these same sources of collagen slightly below the boiling point. Using lower heat allows some, but not all, of the collagen triple helix structure to unwind, resulting in the formation of a characteristic gel upon cooling.

As you know if you have ever made Jell-O from a box, gelatin can be dried, rehydrated in a hot liquid, then chilled, and it will still form a gel. Gelatin differs from a recently developed form of collagen known as hydrolyzed collagen protein, which is gelatin that has enzymatically broken down even further into fragments of proteins called peptides. Hydrolyzed collagen protein will not gel when cooled, but it will dissolve more readily into cold liquids than dried gelatin will.

In China, donkey-hide gelatin, known as *ejiao*, is a very popular remedy by itself or when combined with a variety of Traditional Chinese Medicinal herbs. The first recorded use of ejiao was two thousand years ago, and it continues to be highly valued to this day. On its own, it is believed to confer several health benefits, including increasing overall energy, replenishing blood flow, curing coughs, and treating insomnia. Unfortunately, its popularity, combined with the challenges of raising donkeys on a large enough scale to meet consumer demand, has led to an almost 50 percent reduction in the donkey population in China over the past several years. Note that this is not an endorsement of ejiao—I won't be recommending you consume donkey-hide gelatin. But as you read on, you will see how other types of dietary collagen and gelatin may provide benefits to individuals who experience similar health concerns.

Starting as early as the first century AD, gelatin began to be used as a hemostatic, or blood-stopping, agent in China and Japan. At the end of the eighteenth century, a young medical doctor working in a Paris hospital, Paul Carnot, introduced Western medicine to the use of gelatin as a hemostatic agent. By the 1940s, gelatin foam was being employed in modern hospitals in this way, followed by micro-fibrillar collagen in 1970; both are still in frequent use to this day. Scientists continue researching and developing advanced forms of gelatin/collagen products to effectively stop blood flow, also considering other medical applications, including tissue grafting.

Another long-standing therapeutic use of gelatin has been in the treatment of a variety of digestive disorders. Gelatin forms a hydrophilic colloid, which is basically a water-attracting substance that stays suspended in a liquid. Its many gastrointestinal benefits have been attributed to these properties. Francis Pottenger Jr., a nutrition pioneer in the early twentieth century, reported that when used in conjunction with clinically appropriate dietary modifications, gelatin aided in the digestion of foodstuffs, even foods that may have caused a person difficulty or discomfort after eating. He consistently recommended gelatin-based meals for a wide range of problems, including heartburn, stomach ulcers, spastic colon, and what was then called "nervous digestion," which was accompanied by recurrent vomiting.

Pottenger's contemporaries confirmed his findings, although some attributed the results instead to the ability of gelatin to coat the intestines or its inability to undergo fermentation in the intestines, which often underlies the overgrowth of undesirable bacteria. Today, both holistic medical doctors and nutritionists recommend gelatin-rich broths for patients with gastrointestinal problems. We now recognize that the majority of these problems involve some degree of "gut dysbiosis," or the overgrowth of pathogenic (disease-causing) bacteria and fungi in proportion to the beneficial ones that normally reside in the digestive tract. Although by no means proven, gelatin may interfere with some of this overgrowth while also supporting the digestive process.

Even before collagen and gelatin came into use for medical protocols and in medicinal formulas, they were a significant part of the diet of our earliest ancestors. These "primitive" humans were by necessity very resourceful when it came to using their available food supplies. No part of an animal, whether hunted or raised, went to waste. The bones and tough connective tissues were simmered into stocks that were not only flavorful but also nourishing. After using them for stocks, the bones were ground up using stone tools and then consumed. We now know that besides being excellent sources of calcium and other vital minerals, bones are rich sources of collagen protein. Our ancestors may not have understood the molecular breakdown of what they were eating, but they almost certainly recognized the health value.

Traditional dishes eaten around the globe serve as rich sources of collagen and other important nutrients. In the northern regions of the Arctic, the Inuits rely on a staple dish called *muktuk* made from the skin and blubber of whales. Muktuk is highly nutritious, supplying not only collagen, but also vitamin D and essential fats. In South America, fish heads, which are rich in collagen and other nutrients like vitamin A and iodine, are simmered with vegetables and herbs, creating a base for a soup called *caldillo de congrio*, Spanish for "conger [fish] stock." A globally eaten food dating back to the Middle Ages is headcheese—not a cheese made from milk, but from the head of a pig boiled with the tongue, feet, and heart to create a jellied cold cut.

Oxtail soup is another collagen-rich delicacy that is thought to have originated from French immigrants living in seventeenth-century

England, later adapted as an ethnic dish in the American South, and still very popular in Asian cuisines today. A traditional Vietnamese dish is pho, soup made from a base of collagen-rich bone broth to which a variety of meats and vegetables are added. One of the most popular additions to pho are pieces of beef tendon that have been cooked to the point that they require very little chewing at all. Not only delectable, tendon is about 80 percent collagen protein.

In the late seventeenth century, French physicist Denis Papin invented the earliest form of a pressure cooker, which he named the "digester." Papin hoped his digester could help economically disadvantaged individuals extract more nutrition from bones, but unfortunately, it proved to be much too expensive for the target population. Shortly thereafter, Papin's creation found use on a larger scale to efficiently extract gelatin, considered an extremely nutritious foodstuff, to feed an ever-increasing French population, especially the large numbers of hospital patients and children in orphanages. Philanthropists in Germany and England later set up kitchens that served prepared soups based on gelatin. As with most trends in diet and nutrition, this one went a bit too far: People began to study whether meals consisting solely of gelatin and bread could sustain animals and humans. It quickly became apparent that this type of diet could not sustain life, causing gelatin to fall out of favor.

We now know that although neither gelatin nor collagen protein are sufficient protein sources on their own, their constituent amino acids are nutritionally beneficial to an overall well-balanced diet. And in fact, in the late 1800s, scientist Carl Voit pointed out that gelatin has "protein-sparing" properties, meaning that it can help prevent the breakdown of the body's protein when added to a mixed diet.

Today there is a resurgence of interest in traditionally prepared dishes like the ones mentioned above, both because of their nutritional attributes and because of the growing interest in "nose-to-tail" eating, which utilizes all the parts of an animal. Bone broth and soup stocks made from otherwise discarded animal parts are heralded as nutrition superstars, in part because of the abundant collagen protein they contain.

In my nutrition practice, I encourage patients to incorporate the full gamut of animal products, especially offal (organ meats), skin, and bone broth, into their diets. But if you, like the vast majority of my patients age 40 and younger, grew up eating only skinless and boneless meat, poultry, and fish, perhaps even the thought of eating the "other parts" of an animal leaves you squeamish. If so, you will be glad to know there are ways to obtain the nutritional benefits of collagen that don't require pushing your palate. (While I absolutely love eating pho with tendon and I enjoy a good oxtail soup, not even I have as much as tasted headcheese!) Supplements are one convenient way to get your collagen protein. I'll discuss what to look for when choosing one in Chapter 13.

Increasingly, collagen and collagen-derived products are being utilized in the medical/pharmaceutical, cosmetic, and food industries for both their functional and nutritional properties. Modern studies are backing up what our "primitive ancestors" innately knew and what the first nutritional scientists began to shed light on. Read on so you can be in the know, too!

CHAPTER 3

Why Is Collagen Protein Needed in the Modern-Day Diet?

There are many reasons why we eat, but physiologically, the fundamental purpose is to supply essential nutrients to the almost 40 trillion cells that make up our bodies. (Not to mention to feed those hungry bacteria in our guts that outnumber our own cells by a factor of 10.) Living cells require continuous inputs of both energy (calories) and raw materials (nutrients) for the myriad of biological processes that go on without interruption. That is, until a cell is no longer useful to the body and is selected for death, a process known as apoptosis. When a person is in optimal health, cells that die are immediately replaced by identical cells that will carry on the very same functions.

We must consume enough of the following nutrients regularly to supply the inputs that our cells, and by extension our bodies, absolutely require: carbohydrate and fat for energy; protein; 13 vitamins, 16-plus minerals; a couple of types of essential fats; and water. If even a *single one of these nutrients* is missing or in limited supply, the normal operation of our body can be disrupted. I see this in my nutrition practice daily. Individuals believe they are eating a healthful diet in part by avoiding foods they have heard are bad for their health, yet they're unaware that they may be shortchanging their intake of one or more essential nutrients. In Chapter 14, you will learn about which nutrients to pay attention to when caring for your body's collagen.

Bring up the topic of protein at a gathering of nutritionists and you are almost certain to hear contradictory opinions: "Most people in the United States and other developed countries eat too much protein." "Many people need to increase the amount of protein they eat." "Too much protein is detrimental to bone health." "Inadequate protein intake will lead to a gradual loss of both muscle and bone." "Humans can get all the protein they need from plant sources." "The optimal source of protein is from an animal." Whew—totally not surprising that the public is uncertain on what or who to believe.

The other two macronutrients, fat and carbohydrate, are not without their own controversies. When people ask me what I think about low-carb, low-fat, high-protein diets, I tell them there is no one-size-fits-all nutrition plan. That may sound like I'm dodging the question, but my answer couldn't be any more true. That's why I always create customized macronutrient recommendations for my clients. I believe that in the future, this will be the practice of all dietitians and nutritionists, especially as we gain access to more extensive genomic and metabolic testing.

As far as protein is concerned, we can feel confident of a few facts: Yes, some people eat too much protein, but many people need to eat more. Yes, proteins from animal sources—meat, poultry, seafood, eggs, and dairy—are the proteins with the highest "biological value" and should be included in at least small amounts every day, even when consuming sufficient amounts of plant proteins. Biological value is determined by measuring what proportion of a particular protein, eaten in isolation from other foods, gets incorporated into the proteins of a living organism. Animal-sourced proteins are typically between 75 and 96 percent incorporated into our body's own proteins, with eggs and whey protein topping the list according to biological value.

Another way to understand biological value is how well a protein matches the body's essential amino acid profile. There are nine essential amino acids—histidine, isoleucine, leucine, lysine, methionine, phenylalanine, threonine, tryptophan, and valine—which must be consumed in adequate amounts over the course of the day. Should even just one of these be missing, or present in insufficient quantity, the body will not be able to manufacture the full array of proteins it needs to function. All nine essential amino acids must be present in the right proportions to build the characteristic chains that make up the body's proteins. Interestingly, in isolation, collagen protein has a biological value of zero, due to the absence of tryptophan. But keep reading—collagen will redeem itself!

Most plant sources of protein, such beans and grains, have less than 70 percent biological value when eaten in isolation, with a few exceptions like soybeans and quinoa. This lower number is due to the fact they contain a lesser amount of at least one essential amino acid compared to animal proteins. Since we almost never eat a single protein food all by itself, biological values have somewhat of a limited application, especially since plant proteins can be complementary. For example, grains are low in the amino acid lysine but high in the amino acid methionine, and conversely, legumes are high in lysine but low in methionine. By eating grains and legumes together (such as beans and rice) we in effect fill in many of the gaps, improving the overall protein quality of plant-based foods.

Recall that there are also nonessential amino acids, which are still required for the body to function, but can be made by the body. These include alanine, asparagine, aspartic acid, and glutamic acid. Your body generally has no problem manufacturing these types of amino acids unless you decide to follow an extremely restrictive diet where your overall intake of calories and protein is very low.

There is a third category of amino acids called conditionally essential amino acids: arginine, cysteine, glutamine, tyrosine, glycine, ornithine, proline, and serine. These can be created by the body, but not always in sufficient amounts, depending on the body's overall health status and nutrient needs. During illness and stress, these may become essential, meaning they must be included in the diet for the body to recover effectively.

This last fact gives us another clue into why collagen protein is important for us to consume. Collagen protein is rich in glycine, but most of the other proteins that we eat are not. When we are in good health, our body should be able make plenty of glycine from other amino acids. However, as we shall learn, this does not even occur under optimal conditions.

Glycine, the smallest of all the amino acids, plays a lot of big roles. One of glycine's most important roles is in the healthy turnover of collagen in our bodies. (Turnover simply means the replacement of an older molecule with a newly synthesized one.) Collagen turnover used to be thought of as an extremely slow process, with each collagen molecule having a lifespan of several years.[1] Over the past two decades, this idea has been challenged by studies show-

---

[1] Interestingly, we also know now that the rate of collagen turnover actually speeds up as we get older. This is thought to be due to an increase in "modified collagen," which is more susceptible to the action of collagen-degrading enzymes.

ing that collagen turnover is a very significant portion of the total daily turnover of proteins in our body, representing about one-third of the average daily turnover of 300 grams of the body's protein.[2] Furthermore, we've learned that the rate of collagen renewal is far from static and can be increased with nutritional intakes over and above our minimum needs.

So why is it desirable that our collagen turns over more rapidly? Because the older our collagen is, the more time it has had to undergo undesirable chemical changes. The longer it hangs around without being replaced, the more it becomes oxidized (damaged by oxygen), glycated (attached to blood glucose), and excessively cross-linked. Together, these processes cause our collagen to become stiffer and less flexible, and over time accelerate the "aging" of our bodies.

What can we do to help improve the pace of our collagen turnover? Without question, we must consume an adequate amount of protein, as this affects the turnover of all the proteins in our bodies. When we eat protein-deficient or even protein-marginal diets, our bodies adapt by decreasing overall protein turnover. Strict vegetarians are more likely to experience this because they often eat less protein, and the proteins they eat are typically lower in biological value. Of course, this reduction in protein turnover happens largely imperceptibly, but the cumulative effect can result in a loss of muscle mass, bone strength, and even a reduction in immunity to disease.

Generally, a recommendation of 1 gram of protein per kilogram (roughly 2 pounds) of your body weight is a good place to start. More may be needed if you are very muscular, extremely active, 50 years of age or older, or recovering from an injury or illness.

---

2   We need to eat a lot less than 300 grams (more than 2½ pounds of meat, for example) of protein each day because most of the amino acids from the proteins that are broken down in our bodies are recycled into new proteins.

For a healthy 150-pound woman, 75 grams or more protein is recommended; for a healthy 200-pound man, 100 grams or more is recommended. This does not mean you need large quantities of meat. For example, a 4-ounce serving of beef, chicken, or fish supplies about 30 grams of protein; a cup of cooked legumes supplies about 15 grams; and almost every whole food that we eat supplies at least 1 to 2 grams of protein per typical serving.

Even though the recommended daily totals are not that difficult to reach, a lot of patients who come to see me start out with dietary protein intakes that are less than optimal. You might want to review your own intake to see where you stand; there are several smartphone and computer apps that do this quite well. A few popular ones are MyFitnessPal, SparkPeople, and Lose It!

Just as important as meeting your overall protein needs is meeting your body's need for glycine. You may be thinking, if so many people are suffering from a glycine deficiency, certainly this wouldn't be the only place you would have heard about it. While this is not breaking news, I believe you would be surprised to learn that most people could significantly benefit from additional glycine in their diet. A group of scientists from Spain and France concluded this very thing, stating, "Nutritional and clinical studies during the past 20 years indicate that *the amount of glycine available in humans is not enough to meet metabolic needs and that a dietary supplement is appropriate.*" (Emphasis mine.)

To come to this conclusion, these scientists began with the established fact that the typical diet supplies between 1.5 and 3 grams of glycine daily, depending on the quantity as well as the quality of the protein consumed by a given individual. They then determined that the human body produces about 3 grams of glycine per day, mainly from the amino acid serine, with lesser contributions from other dietary precursors. This adds up to between 4.5 and 6 grams of glycine being supplied daily. The scientists then added up the needs the body has for glycine, predominantly for the synthesis of collagen, the antioxidant glutathione, bile to digest fats, the heme group in hemoglobin (which transports oxygen), and a few other biological processes; this totaled to about 14.5 grams per day. By far, the greatest demand for glycine was for collagen synthesis, requiring about 12 grams per day to fully maximize turnover.

The scientists calculated the difference between the supply of and the demand for glycine, determining that there is an average shortfall of between 8.5 and 10 grams per day. Is this a meaningful shortfall, and if so, what problems can arise over time?

Two particularly critical periods when a glycine shortfall has deleterious effects are during pregnancy and the senior years of life. We'll cover these life stages in more detail in Chapter 11. A glycine shortage is somewhat less serious for the average person under the age of 60, but it is still problematic. As already mentioned, the turnover of our own collagen decreases proportionately along with a deficit of glycine, accelerating the pace of damage in every tissue rich in collagen. And, as we'll see from studies in later chapters, when we eat collagen protein, we are able to refresh the parts of our bodies that are full of collagen. Topping off our glycine pool is one important reason consuming collagen protein helps us make more collagen.

A seemingly small amount of glycine, 2.5 grams, is needed to meet all our other needs beyond the synthesis of collagen. But those other needs are extremely important. For example, without enough glycine, there can be a decreased production of glutathione. Glutathione is known as the body's "master antioxidant," an impressive title for sure. Studies indicate that glycine deficiencies result in an increase in the rate of damaging oxidative stress on the body. This and other special roles for glycine are reviewed in Chapter 10.

Proline may be almost as important to pay attention to as glycine. Proline, together with a modified form of proline called hydroxyproline, comprises about one-quarter of the amino acids in collagen protein. Furthermore, we need more proline than other amino acids when it comes to whole-body protein synthesis.

Proline is also a major starting material in the body's synthesis of arginine, an amino acid needed to produce an important molecule called nitric oxide. Nitric oxide is involved in the regulation of blood flow, the contraction of muscles, and the transport of nutrients, among other roles. It acts as a natural vasodilator, meaning it widens the blood vessels to permit blood to flow optimally to all parts of the body. If you consider yourself an athlete, you may already be familiar with nitric oxide for its ability to help enhance exercise performance. And with arginine making up 9 percent of collagen protein, even more reason for athletes to love it!

Like glycine, our bodies make proline from other amino acids, including dietary arginine (proline and arginine convert to each other as the body demands). But in experiments where individuals were fed proline-free diets, the levels of proline in their blood dropped by 20 to 30 percent, confirming that dietary proline is required to optimize the body's levels of proline. How much is needed is still not fully quantified.

Unlike glycine, almost all foods rich in protein are also good sources of proline, but the best sources are collagen protein (23 percent proline and hydroxyproline) and milk proteins (12 percent proline). It makes sense that milk is rich in proline—newborns have a high need for proline that exceeds their capacity to synthesize it in the early stages of life. It may be difficult to obtain enough proline from your diet if you are a strict vegan, as animal proteins in general contain three to six times greater amounts of proline than plant proteins.

Assuming that a diet is adequate in protein, the more common problem is likely to be a shortage of hydroxyproline rather than proline. Hydroxyproline must be made by our bodies from the proline in our diets, a process that requires both vitamin C and iron. Hydroxyproline is needed along with a second "hydroxylated" amino acid, hydroxylysine, to form procollagen, the precursor to our body's collagen. Ideally, vitamin C-rich food should be eaten daily to support this ongoing process.

During wound healing it is especially important to consume foods rich in proline, as the body needs extra proline to repair damaged tissue. We'll delve into all of the important roles for proline in Chapter 10.

Collagen Protein: More Than Just the Sum of Its Parts

Collagen protein acts in ways that go well beyond the effects of its individual amino acids. Each chapter of this book is devoted to a different benefit you could see from consuming collagen protein.

But before launching into what makes collagen protein so exciting, you should understand some simple terminology I will be using throughout this book. First, I will use the generic term "collagen protein" to mean any of the various types of dietary collagen protein: purified gelatin, intact sources like poultry skin and beef tendon, and collagen peptides. When I use the word "collagen" by itself, it will specifically refer to the collagen we have in our own bodies.

Next, you need to understand the basic difference between collagen protein in the form of gelatin and collagen protein in the form of collagen peptides.

Gelatin is a *partially broken-down* form of collagen protein. It is obtained by first treating a source of animal collagen protein (skin, bones, scales, etc.) with either an acid or base, followed by heating it until the individual strands of animal collagen protein separate from each other. The earliest scientific studies on collagen protein used gelatin, because hydrolyzed collagen protein, discussed next, has only been available for about a decade. Gelatin especially benefits nails and digestive health, as does bone broth that contains gelatin and other nutritious substances. Gelatin has the special property of congealing into a gel because it is only partially broken-down, retaining the hydrogen atoms that are responsible for it attracting water.

But what you may be predominantly seeing on store shelves and all over the internet is what I will consistently refer to as "collagen peptides," unless I am discussing the details of a study, and then I will use the specific terminology that the authors used. The familiar terms "collagen peptides," "hydrolyzed collagen," and "collagen hydrolysate," and the less often used "hydrolyzed gelatin," all refer to the same product: collagen protein that has been *more completely broken down* into smaller pieces through the use of special protein-digesting enzymes. The term "hydrolyzed collagen peptides" is occasionally used, but it is redundant, as all peptide forms of collagen have been hydrolyzed.

If you are still a bit confused about what the differences are, there are just a few things you need to keep in mind. One, collagen peptides are the focus of almost all the current research and for good reason, as you'll find out. Two, it is thought that the presence of "bioactive" dipeptides and tripeptides (two–amino acid units and three–amino acid units, respectively) in collagen peptide products is the reason for many of their health benefits. And three, the degree of and specificity of the hydrolysis, or how much and which active dipeptide and tripeptides a collagen product contains, can vary.

What makes collagen peptides so special? While it used to be thought that all proteins and peptides were completely broken down into their constituent amino acids (e.g., glycine and proline) in the digestive tract, we now know that this is not the case. There are several collagen dipeptides and tripeptides that bypass complete digestion, leaving as many as 10 percent remaining intact as they enter the bloodstream. These bioactive peptides continue to circulate for several hours. From the blood, they are transferred to the many places, such as the skin and joints, where they can continue to exert their beneficial effects for up to two weeks. Most of these bioactive peptides contain hydroxyproline, which is mainly connected to proline but also to other amino acids.

Our own gastrointestinal tract may also generate bioactive peptides due to the fact that, similar to other dietary proteins, intact collagen protein resists complete digestion. However, there are no published studies indicating how much is produced and whether the amount produced exerts the same beneficial effects as supplemental collagen peptides. The consensus in the literature is that the amount made from dietary sources of intact collagen protein (as opposed to collagen peptides) is too small to induce any meaningful effects. On the other hand, people who regularly include foods rich in collagen protein self-report that their skin and joints respond favorably. It is plausible that the process of simmering bones for an extended period of time may yield some active collagen peptides in addition to intact gelatin.

In the chapters that follow, I'll be presenting some of the best research available so you can decide which method of consuming collagen protein is right for you. We'll start with what a lot of women and men want to know—does collagen protein really deliver the beauty benefits it promises?

CHAPTER 4

Beauty from Within

Smooth, glowing, even-toned, youthful-looking skin—is there any more sought-after physical asset? People of all ages, races, and genders want it. The market for anti-aging skin products has exploded—in 2016, sales in the U.S. alone exceeded $1 billion. Many people begin using anti-aging products before they even turn 30, hoping to stay ahead of the lines, uneven pigmentation, and loss of firmness that seem to accelerate with each decade of life. And right up there with our collective love of skin care products is our national obsession with thick, shiny hair and fingernails.

Looking good helps us make great first impressions and can really boost our self-confidence. And if we take good care of ourselves, our appearance can belie our real age. A youthful appearance is more than just physical attractiveness—it is a window into overall health and vitality. While creams and lotions and other topical treatments can help, one of the best ways to stay young-looking on the outside is to stay young on the inside!

In this chapter you will learn how dietary collagen can help support the health of the integumentary system. Medically speaking, the integumentary system is the term for the organ system consisting of the skin, the single largest organ in our body, and two accessory structures, the nails and hair. Together, this trio creates a barrier to the outside world, protecting us from physical, chemical, microbial, and radiation exposures. Equally important, the integumentary system functions to regulate our body heat and moisture by continually sensing and adjusting to the changing environment around us.

Our Largest Organ

The largest organ in our body, skin contains 40 percent of our body's collagen protein. Skin is the easiest place to evaluate the overall state of our body's collagen, especially in areas that have largely been protected from sun exposure. Take a look at your skin closely: Is it dull or radiant? Does it have a warm color or is it tending toward a dull gray? Is it mostly firm or are you beginning to notice sagging in areas such as around your jawline and your eyes? Do you feel you have more or fewer lines and age spots than others your age? Do you have an excessive amount of stretch marks or perhaps cellulite (much more likely if you are a woman)? All of these changes are to some extent normal, but if you feel you might be aging more rapidly than you should be, it's never too late to take action!

Many factors determine how our skin matures and ages. Our genetic makeup will govern the rate to some extent, yet we all know families where the elder sibling looks years younger than his or her juniors. Ultraviolet light, smoking, insufficient exercise, air pollution and other toxins, too little sleep, and fluctuations in body weight all contribute to a more rapid decline in the youthful appearance of the skin. Sun exposure is the main cause of ultraviolet-induced photoaging, thought to be the biggest factor under our control. Photoaging is an acceleration of the normal aging of the skin due to the penetration of ultraviolet light into the deeper layers of the skin, degrading the skin's collagen and then interfering with the rebuilding of the damaged collagen. Next to this, eating a nourishing diet rich in collagen protein ranks right up there in the things we can do for our skin.

Before we delve into the studies that demonstrate how a diet rich in collagen impacts skin, a short review of the anatomy and physiology of the skin can provide some background. Skin is composed of three interconnected and interdependent layers: the epidermis, or thinner outermost layer; the dermis, the thicker inner layer that gives the skin its strength and elasticity; and the hypodermis, a cushiony, fat-rich layer of tissue beneath the dermis.

The epidermis is made up of either four or five layers of cells, 90 percent of which are rich in the protein keratin, hence their name, keratinocytes. Keratin differs from collagen in a number of ways, explained at the end of this chapter. The outermost layer of keratinocytes is so far removed from the underlying dermis that these cells continuously die off from a lack of nutrients, shedding at a rate of approximately 40,000 cells per minute. If you have ever wondered where so much dust in your home comes from, a lot of it is just dead skin cells! These sloughed-off cells are constantly being replaced by brand-new keratinocytes arriving from the underlying layers. Other cells residing in the epidermis include melanocytes, which produce the skin pigment melanin, and Langerhans cells, which fight off disease-causing microbes.

The dermis is directly under the epidermis and has two layers. One layer borders the epidermis, just reaching into it with finger-like projections. These projections supply nutrients and oxygen to the epidermis and contain nerves that allow us to sense touch, temperature, and pain through the surface of our skin. The second, deeper layer of the dermis is made primarily from large-diameter collagen fibers that are organized into bundles and wrapped with elastin-containing fibers, making up the connective tissue that forms the majority of our skin. Unlike the epidermis, the dermis does not completely replace itself, which is why our skin color and texture generally remains the same throughout our lives.

Type I collagen is the most abundant collagen in the dermis, organized into fibrils that interconnect to create larger collagen fibers. The size and arrangement of the type I collagen fibrils determine the mechanical and the physical properties of the skin. In addition, the basement membrane, the thin layer between the epidermis and dermis, contains about 50 percent type IV collagen, which forms the cross-linked network and creates stability.

Below the dermis lies a layer of loose connective tissue called the hypodermis. This is where we find our "subcutaneous adipose tissue," or the fat just below our skin that keeps us warm, provides cushioning over muscles and bones, and helps mold our body contours. Far from being inert, subcutaneous fat is a metabolically active region of the body, playing a role in both blood sugar and cholesterol regulation. Compared to the fat located within our abdominal region (visceral fat), subcutaneous fat is coming to be understood as a beneficial type of fat deposit.

What Happens to Skin as We Get Older?

Several undesirable changes occur to our skin as we age: It gradually becomes thinner, loses subcutaneous fat, and overall looks less plump and smooth than during our youth. Scratches, cuts, or burns take longer to heal. Collagen is one of the major components of the skin that is responsible for its condition and appearance, but unfortunately, both the amount and the density of collagen in the skin decreases with age and exposure to damaging ultraviolet light.

In addition, the highly organized collagen network in the dermis layer becomes increasingly less organized as we age, a process called fragmentation. Fragmentation causes the bundles of collagen fibrils to become looser, thinner, and shorter, leading to a reduction in dermal thickness. As these disorganized collagen fibrils separate from the surrounding fibroblasts, even more fragmentation occurs. This self-perpetuating process is not just limited to chronological aging; excessive UV exposure causes a virtually identical process.

On a molecular level, a group of enzymes called "matrix photoaging metalloproteinases" heavily accounts for rapid collagen degradation. To greatly simplify, escalating activity of metalloproteinases causes the collagen fibrils to become more and more fragmented. Then the fibroblasts lose their sites of attachment on collagen. With the loss of binding sites, the fibroblasts are no longer maintained in their naturally stretched state. This leads to still more metalloproteinase activity and less collagen production.

Unfortunately, metalloproteinases are not only found in the skin, but anywhere there is an abundance of collagen: bone, cartilage, tendons, and ligaments. And although this process is impossible to prevent, exposure to UV rays does two things: It speeds up the metalloproteinase activity and suppresses collagen synthesis even more. So while pretty much your whole body is affected over time, your skin is most vulnerable to this process. In fact, much of skin's aging is due to repeated sun exposure.

These aging processes proceed more rapidly with each decade of life, slowly but surely causing the skin to first develop fine lines, followed by superficial wrinkles, and finally deeper wrinkles and drooping, especially around the mouth, jawline, and eyes. For women, the changes start to become very noticeable after meno-pause, on not only the face, but also other exposed parts of the body, like the neck and upper chest. Men generally experience a steadier decline in their skin's appearance with age.

As we age, there is a slow and steady decline in the amount of hyaluronic acid in both the dermis and epidermis, simultaneous to the breakdown of collagen. Hyaluronic acid is the skin's natural hydrator, able to hold up to 1,000 times its weight in water. The gradual loss of hyaluronic acid is reflected in the skin's reduced capacity to retain moisture, so skin becomes drier with age. Dry skin is visually undesirable because it magnifies the appearance of lines and wrinkles and makes the skin appear rough. Dryness is also unhealthy because it impairs the protective function of the epidermis.

How to Take Action with Collagen

A good sunblock is your best friend when it comes to keeping your skin youthful. After that, you can choose from a variety of topical youth serums and creams. We won't discuss which ingredients to look for because that would be a whole other book! But while we're on the subject, you might be curious to know if the surface of the skin can absorb collagen. Collagen protein is an ingredient in a variety of cosmetic creams and lotions, despite limited evidence that it delivers results. The only type of topically applied collagen that may potentially offer benefits is one that has been hydrolyzed into very small peptides, but this may cause a risk for allergic dermatitis in some people. One study showed that four weeks of applying a *synthetic* collagen-like peptide reduced wrinkling around the eyes in women ages 40 to 62. I could only identify one manufacturer that provided collagen peptides for cosmetic applications that were both safe and effective (BioCell Collagen CG-WS), but no products are yet available to consumers in the United States.

For optimal skin health, good nutrition is absolutely essential; studies on a wide range of nutrients and foods have repeatedly proven this. And a diet that is rich in collagen protein is one of the best ways to feed the skin, helping it stay moister, firmer, smoother, and less reactive to environmental insults.

Before we look at some of the studies, you might be curious to know how actually consuming collagen protein works to help the skin stay more youthful. You learned in Chapter 3 what happens when hydrolyzed collagen peptides are ingested—a significant amount passes through the intestines and remains intact as it enters the blood stream. Some then gets stored in tissues like cartilage and skin. But what happens after this may surprise you as it did me.

One current understanding is that these circulating peptides send a *false* signal that existing collagen is actively being destroyed. This in turn leads to an increase in the synthesis of brand-new, stronger collagen protein fibrils. Simultaneously, these collagen peptides stimulate the synthesis of hyaluronic acid, responsible for holding moisture in the skin. Additionally, collagen peptides decrease the overactivity of the matrix metalloproteinases that cause the breakdown of the collagen in our bodies.

Beginning with pre-clinical studies on isolated tissues and with laboratory animals, and progressing to clinical studies with human volunteers, scientists have been examining what happens when collagen proteins are added to the tissue growth media or the diet. A major goal is to find out what works to increase skin moisture and reduce lines, wrinkling, sagging, roughness, and discoloration. These are the same things we all want to know, so let's see what they learned.

We'll start with the most intriguing research—the clinical studies that look at what happens when real people consume collagen protein on a daily basis. The majority of the studies on skin were conducted on women, probably because women have traditionally been more concerned than men with the appearance of their skin (women can't hide behind a beard!). However, that doesn't mean the results don't apply to guys as well.

Retaining Moisture in the Skin

In a three-part study published in the *Journal of Cosmetic Dermatology* in 2015, one research group conducted two clinical trials using collagen peptides, the first with Japanese women, the second with French women. In the third trial, the scientists measured the changes in tiny samples of human skin following incubation with collagen peptides.

In the first clinical trial, 33 healthy Japanese women ages 40 to 59 participated. They were pre-selected due to the low water content of their skin. They were divided into three parallel groups, evenly distributed according to the participant's skin water content, and given a drink formulated with 10 grams of a placebo (dextrin) or with 10 grams of one of two collagen peptides, either of fish or porcine origin (Peptan F or Peptan P). The women were told to consume their drink at bedtime; no instructions on skin care were given. After four and eight weeks of treatment, the women's facial skin was analyzed for moisture content and rate of water loss using specialized electronic devices.

The group who consumed Peptan F had a 12 percent increase in skin moisture after the full eight weeks, but even more exciting were the results in the Peptan P group. These women had a 16 percent increase in moisture at the four-week midpoint, and as much as a

28 percent increase in eight weeks! There was no difference in the rate of water loss among the three groups, signifying that all the increased moisture was being generated from within the skin. (I'll explain what is behind this increase when I discuss the third study from this publication, on page 42.)

Restoring moisture to dry skin—how many serums, lotions, and creams promise to do just that? It is true that some topical products perform better than others in preventing the *loss* of skin hydration. But elevating the water content generated from within the skin is key, and this study shows that dietary collagen protein can do just that! It is too early to conclude that collagen peptides from a porcine source (pigs) have the most hydrating potential, but this could prove to be the case. Pig skin is used in treating massive burns and injuries and in healing persistent skin ulcers, because pigs' skin is most similar to ours. (Note that keeping the humidity in your home above 30 percent, taking shorter and cooler showers, and drinking plenty of fluids are also effective strategies for preventing skin dehydration.)

In the second clinical trial, 99 French women ages 40 to 65 were randomly split into two groups and given a powdered drink mix containing either 10 grams of a placebo (maltodextrin, also known as food starch) or 10 grams of fish collagen peptides (Peptan F). The women consumed their assigned beverage each morning before breakfast. They were instructed not to use beauty care products or get more than casual sun exposure for the duration of the 12-week study. At the end of the 12 weeks, the group who consumed the Peptan F collagen showed a 9 percent increase in overall collagen density and a 31 percent decrease in the fragmentation of the collagen in the dermis layer of their skin, which was measured on their forearms with high-frequency ultrasound.

Improvements were noted just four weeks after they began consuming the Peptan F collagen and were still visible 12 weeks after the women had stopped this morning routine. In just three months of daily collagen peptide consumption, women in this second trial showed a significant increase in collagen synthesis in their skin. Perhaps even more exciting, this is the first clinical study to show that the detrimental process of collagen fragmentation can be significantly reversed by the consumption of collagen peptides.

This study was not long enough to compare the changes in the two groups' appearances over an extended period of time, as this type of study would be prohibitively expensive to conduct. However, it is reasonable to conclude that including collagen protein in your daily diet long-term would continue to enhance your skin's ability to fight the ravages of aging.

The third study was somewhat different from the first two as it was conducted using tiny samples of skin tissue obtained from the thigh of a 49-year-old woman. These samples were placed into a liquid medium to which increasing amounts of fish collagen peptides (Peptan F) were added. After incubating for nine days, the skin samples were removed and examined under a microscope. The scientists observed an increase in the collagen content that reached a maximum of 9 percent. In addition, they observed a 17-fold increase in the skin's glycosaminoglycan content.

Glycosaminoglycans are a diverse class of molecule, consisting of long chains of repeating pairs of carbohydrates. They strongly attract and bind water in the skin and other places like the joints and the mucus-producing linings in the gut. You've already learned about one very important type of glycosaminoglycan, hyaluronic acid, which attracts and holds water in the skin. While a 17-fold increase measured from a skin sample doesn't necessarily translate to a real person's skin, an increase in glycosaminoglycan content could explain the results of the first study. Women who consumed the collagen peptides experienced a 12 to 28 percent elevation in the overall moisture content of their skin in less than two months' time.

Reducing Wrinkles

Another clinical trial was published in 2013 in the journal *Skin Pharmacology and Physiology*. In this study, 144 female volunteers ages 45 to 65 participated in one of two treatment groups, taking either 2.5 grams of a placebo or the same amount of a bioactive collagen peptide (Verisol, manufactured in Germany), both in the form of a powder to be dissolved daily into a liquid of their choosing. These women were told not to use any leave-on skin care or makeup products and to avoid getting more than casual UV or sun exposure.

Changes in skin wrinkling were quantified using software that performs 3D matching, which compared before and after images of the outer corners of the women's eyes. After four weeks of treatment, the women consuming the collagen peptides had a greater than 7 percent reduction in eye wrinkle volume compared to the placebo group; after eight weeks, their wrinkle volume decreased an average of 20 percent, with some women showing an almost 50 percent reduction. The positive effects on their skin persisted even four weeks after stopping the collagen. Interestingly, the wrinkle volume in the placebo group actually worsened by 15 percent after eight weeks, potentially due to changes in climatic conditions that equally affected both groups.

In addition to measuring skin surface changes, the researchers drew fluids from the women's forearms through a procedure called suction blistering. In the collagen peptide group, as compared to the placebo, the fluids drawn contained 65 percent more procollagen and 18 percent more elastin. As explained earlier, collagen and elastin are the major components in the dermis layer that support skin elasticity and firmness. The increases in these levels were suggested as the reason for the long-lasting reductions in wrinkle volume even after the collagen peptides were discontinued.

In a previously published study using the Verisol brand of bioactive collagen peptide, these same researchers demonstrated a significant improvement in skin elasticity in female volunteers 35 to 55 years of age. A couple of things were interesting about this earlier study. One, there was no additional improvement in elasticity in the women who were given 5 grams as compared to 2.5 grams of collagen peptide daily. And two, the most pronounced improvement occurred in the women who were over 50, confirming that it is never too late to get on board with collagen protein!

Verisol is one of several bovine-derived collagen peptides available in the United States and other countries. It is manufactured by Gelita, whose German plant is the world's largest producer of collagen peptides. It appears to be a well-reviewed product, and it gives maximum results in just 2.5 grams (or 2500 mg) taken daily. Verisol is available as an ingredient in a variety of flavored and unflavored products including ones sold by Whole Foods, Life Extension, and Country Life, as well as the German company Besha. Beyond skin improvement, some regular users report that their hair and nails grow faster and thicker, and they notice an improvement in the appearance of cellulite.

Be sure to read the label carefully before you purchase Verisol or any other collagen product, as it may contain additional ingredients that you need to avoid or do not want to consume. Conversely, some products add in other nutrients like hyaluronic acid, herbal extracts, and vitamins and minerals that do support skin, nail, and hair health (more on this in Chapter 14). Note that Verisol collagen does not necessarily claim to be a pasture-raised or a non-GMO product, if that is important to you (see Chapter 13).

These two research reports are important because they both included placebo groups and because neither the scientists nor the participants knew in advance which participants were given placebo or collagen protein. These types of studies, called randomized double-blind placebo-controlled trials, are the gold standard in clinical research. They minimize bias and allow for comparisons to be made with better confidence. The scientists also used electronic and computerized equipment to measure the results and make comparisons, rather than relying on subjective outcomes such as measuring the degree of wrinkling with the unaided human eye.

Help Banish Those Annoying Spots

While there is minimal published data on the effect of collagen protein on age spots, a study published in 2012 in the *Health Sciences Journal* from Japan is promising. Thirty-nine women, between ages 35 to 50, were divided into three groups and given 5 grams per day of either fish collagen hydrolysate, porcine collagen hydrolysate, or maltodextrin as a placebo. Using a skin imaging testing machine called VISIA II, their faces were examined for changes in melanin (skin pigment), pores, speckles (small patches of color different from the normal skin tone), ultraviolet spots (age spots caused by UV light), wrinkles, and redness.

After eight weeks, the women in the placebo group had no changes in any of these characteristics. The women in both the fish and pig collagen groups experienced a significant decline in age spots on their faces. Of the two types of collagen tested, only the porcine collagen yielded measurable results at four weeks. It also surpassed the results of the fish collagen at the end of the eight-week trial. The researchers determined that the collagen hydrolysates modulated the dermis and epidermis, thus reducing age spots, and the researchers point out the obvious need for a larger study to confirm these findings.

After I reviewed the available data myself, there appeared to be a trend to a reduction in visible pores and redness when consuming collagen peptides. However, the reductions were still small enough that they may have been normal variations due to chance. Pore size is considered for the most part permanent. Currently, laser treatments are the only thing that can make pores physically shrink, due in part to a targeted stimulation of collagen production. Persistent skin redness can have a myriad of causes—inflammation, infection, and superficial capillaries—and can also be medically treated.

If you have age spots or enlarged pores, or your problems with redness are purely cosmetic in nature, my suggestion is to try an experiment yourself. Consume at least half of your daily collagen from a porcine source and be sure to limit your sun exposure to avoid affecting your results. Be sure to take close-up before and after photos for comparison.

Acne

Far more than just a cosmetic concern, acne can really mess with your psyche and self-confidence. Hormones, stress, diet—they all factor in. But bring up the subject of nutrition with a dermatologist and they are likely to tell you that dietary changes will make little if any difference. As a nutritionist, I have witnessed that this is far from the case. Eliminating poor-quality fats (bye-bye, French fries and chips), cutting back on sugar, and replacing processed foods with whole foods can definitely lead to improvements in acne. Making sure the diet provides adequate vitamin A and zinc is important, too, as they can prevent an excessive buildup of keratin that blocks off pores. Last, but certainly not least, is consuming a source of collagen protein on a daily basis.

Will collagen protein work for you to prevent breakouts and heal past acne damage? As of the printing of this book, there are no published research studies on collagen protein's effects on acne. But, since there is little downside to consuming collagen protein, I say, go for it! Start slow, with a quarter of the label dose per day, and gradually increase to the full dose. Give it at least one to two months' time, and please don't ignore the rest of your nutrition, as collagen protein works best in the context of a balanced diet. I did come across a few reviews written by people who said their acne got worse while they were taking collagen protein. This could be due to an enhanced level of detoxification from the glycine (see Chapter 10). If so, this should go away with time. Starting with a lower dose may help minimize this reaction, if it occurs.

Cellulite — Can Anything Be Done?

Just 15 percent of adult women do not have cellulite on their bodies, meaning that the overwhelming majority of women do. If you have cellulite, you are definitely not entirely to blame. Genetic factors, ethnicity, pregnancy, age, and female hormones make women more likely to develop orange peel–textured thighs, buttocks, and bellies. On the other hand, there are a few lifestyle habits that contribute to a worsening of cellulite, namely being overweight, staying sedentary, and eating a poor diet (perhaps one without enough collagen protein).

BEAUTY SLEEP

A predominant amino acid in collagen protein, glycine, has been shown to help the body enter into a deeper state of sleep. Sleep is the critical time for skin regeneration because it is during deep sleep that the majority of our growth hormone is secreted, renewing our body through the natural process of cell division. Indeed, there truly is such a thing as "beauty sleep"! More on this special effect of glycine in Chapter 10.

Cellulite is recognized as a natural process, not a disease, but in severe cases, it can negatively impact quality of life. It is often little consolation that cellulite has a good side: maximizing the storage of fat to ensure plenty of calories are available for pregnancy and breastfeeding. This stubborn condition is characterized by an excess of subcutaneous fat that bulges into the dermis of the skin due to a disordered and weakened underlying structure. Because of this, the goal of any lasting treatment should be to improve dermal strength and density, even as fat stores decline.

Like many women, you may have tried a variety of things to diminish the appearance of cellulite, perhaps without much success. Medically, laser treatments are often helpful, for similar reasons that they are effective in reducing facial pore size. Weight loss can reduce the severity of cellulite but it may not have much impact on the degree of surface dimpling in women who are obese. Massage will temporarily reduce the appearance of cellulite, as it causes fluids to drain away, and it can offer longer-lasting effects due to its stimulation of fibroblast and keratinocyte activity. A few topical products have been studied, as well. A particularly effective one contained black pepper, orange peel, ginger, cinnamon, capsaicin, green tea, and caffeine. It was applied daily under compression shorts and yielded noticeable results in just four weeks..

Where does collagen protein fit into an anti-cellulite game plan? As of the publication of this book, there was just one study that looked at collagen's effects on cellulite. In this clinical trial, 97 women between 25 and 50 years of age consumed either 2.5 grams of collagen peptides (Verisol brand) or a placebo daily, mixing their assigned powder into a beverage of their choosing. After six months, the women in the collagen peptide group with a normal body mass index (less than or equal to 25) displayed a statistically significant 9 percent reduction in the appearance of cellulite, an accompanying 11 percent decrease in the waviness of their thigh skin, and a significant strengthening of their dermal density.

Women in the collagen group who had higher body mass indexes showed fewer improvements that did not reach the level of statistical significance. Because of their higher amounts of body fat, it may be that these women would only see a significant improvement in cellulite appearance after a longer duration of treatment with collagen peptides. There was no mention of weight changes occurring over the course of the study, so it is also possible that the overweight women may have seen better improvements in cellulite appearance if they were given weight-reducing diets along with the collagen protein supplements.

You may want to add a rich source of polyphenols (plant-derived antioxidants) along with your daily collagen peptides to enhance your results. One to try is chokeberry; 3 ounces of this polyphenol-packed juice per day over three months improved the appearance of cellulite by significantly reducing subcutaneous tissue thickness and fluid accumulation. Adding in gotu kola, an herb that promotes lymphatic drainage and exerts other positive effects (see Chapter 14), may additionally improve the appearance of cellulite over time.

My suggestion is to try collagen peptides first, incorporate foods rich in polyphenols into your diet (such as dark-colored berries, pomegranates, olives, green tea, cocoa, and even spices like cloves), then perhaps apply a topical cream like the one tested in the study discussed above if you want to try to accelerate your results.

Nails and Hair

Keratin is the primary component of hair and nails. The protein is similar to collagen in that it consists of three strands of amino acid chains that are twisted into a triple helix and stabilized by cross-links. However, keratin's amino acid sequence is quite different from collagen's. In addition, the cross-links are much stronger in keratin than in collagen. Although our nails and hair do not contain collagen, supplementation with collagen protein has been shown to help them grow.

Nails

Stronger nails mean longer nails because strong nails are naturally more resistant to breaking, chipping, splitting, and peeling. Unfortunately, more than one in four women and one in seven men suffer from weak, fragile nails (not surprisingly, women are more frustrated with their nails' appearance). And because breaking and splitting can expose the nail bed, fragile nails often result in pain. In the absence of a disease, mechanical and chemical damage suffered during the course of daily activities is a chief cause of nail weakening that ultimately leads to breakage. A healthy nail bed has a water content of about 18 percent, and as it drops below 16 percent, the nail weakens. Alternating contact with water followed by drying increases the brittleness of nails, and women seem to be more affected by this process than men, even with similar exposure. Housework is clearly not compatible with growing stronger nails—rubber gloves, anyone?

Women have been on a quest for beautiful nails since ancient times, where vibrant colors signified higher socioeconomic rankings. Modern nail polishes had their start with products inspired by automobile paint in the early twentieth century. The first use of collagen protein, in the form of gelatin, to strengthen nails goes back to the 1950s. If you were a teenage girl or perhaps a young woman around that time, you probably recall the advertisements for Knox Gelatin promising to grow beautiful nails.

A small study conducted in 1949 may have been responsible for launching the Knox Gelatin craze. A medical doctor in New York City followed a dozen patients who had all complained of soft, peeling, and easily broken fingernails. None had an obvious dietary deficiency or a disease of the nail bed. After 13 weeks of consuming 7 grams of gelatin daily, 10 of the 12 saw their nails become normal in firmness. Several also reported improvements in their toenails and in the growth of the hair on their head and their eyebrows. While the written report was only one page in length, there were impressive before and after photos of the hand of one patient who grew beautiful nails despite having been previously plagued with extremely brittle nails.

This preliminary study was followed by a larger one conducted with 82 medical clinic patients; they consumed 7 grams of gelatin daily for 120 days. Doctors took photos twice a month and microscopically examined nail clippings to measure changes in nail growth and structure. Under the microscope, they observed that brittle nails appeared to contain less collagen between the structural layers of keratin. At the end of the trial, 86 percent of patients with brittle nails, even chronically brittle nails, experienced improvements that lasted up to three months after stopping the gelatin. The doctors noted that even in cases where photos did not indicate changes had occurred, patients insisted their nails felt stronger, looked smoother and shinier, and that they could pick up things without them hurting, effects the camera could not capture.

Interestingly, this report mentions the most common dietary cause of brittle nails to be calcium deficiency. I recall learning this same thing early on in my undergraduate education. However, despite adequate calcium intake, it is clear that many people, and especially women, still suffer from nails that break, crack, peel, and split.

Fast-forward to recently published studies on the effects of collagen protein on fingernail quality. In a placebo-controlled study of 20 female volunteers ages 31 to 51 who experienced problems with nail fragility, the group consuming 5 grams per day of porcine-derived collagen peptides had an increase in both the moisture and lipid levels in their fingernails. These improvements resulted in greater nail "suppleness" and flexibility, making them more resistant to breakage.

Another recent study reported decreases in cracked and chipped nails noticeable after only two months of supplementing with the Gelita brand of collagen peptides (Verisol). There was a maximum decrease of 42 percent in cracking and chipping after the full six months of supplementation. In addition, there was a statistically significant increase in the rate of nail growth. The majority of the women in this study said they were "completely satisfied" and perceived their nails to be longer.

Nowadays, there is always the option of creating artificially long and strong fingernails by coating them with one of a variety of acrylic or gel products. My own lifelong frustration with short, brittle nails led me to doing this for almost five years. But I just recently decided to give up my nail salon habit and allow my nails to go *au natural*, something that should be done at least periodically according to the American Academy of Dermatology. It's too early to tell how my own nails will withstand my cooking, gardening, and athletic activities, since I still have a half-inch of damage that needs to grow out. But I already notice that they have a nice pink color, which may signify that the circulation to my nail beds has improved since I've embarked on my own collagen protein regimen just six months ago. This may be one of the ways that collagen and gelatin proteins enhance nail strength—by increasing blood flow to the fingers.

My daughter recently shared with me how happy she was with the results she was seeing from her regular consumption of bovine collagen peptides. Her nails were growing long even though she too had stopped applying gel nail polish. Like me, she had never had naturally long and strong fingernails, so this is quite a remarkable change.

Of my patients who have been consuming collagen protein and/or bone broths on a regular basis, most remark that they see positive changes in their skin, and many tell me that their nails grow faster and stronger. From a scan of numerous online reviews of various collagen products, improvements in nails are noted by about 2 in 10 people. It stands to reason that only those who don't use topically applied gels and hardeners would be able to notice these changes.

For those who are reluctant to give up instantly perfect nails (as I was!), my best advice would be to let one nail, perhaps a pinky finger, grow out. Then watch how that nail responds to daily collagen protein supplementation and decide if you want to bare all 10. You can always go back to the salon, but may discover that you can better use the time for truly health-promoting habits like exercise or a massage.

Hair

Like our nails, our hair consists mainly of the protein keratin. Unlike our nails, however, after our hair grows out of the scalp, it no longer receives nourishment from the blood vessels. Knowing this, I was planning to skip the topic of hair and collagen protein entirely. But then I came across some manufacturers' claims that their collagen protein product can moisturize dry hair, reduce graying, and even repair split ends, which seemed too good to be true. I was still skeptical about any role collagen protein would have in hair health and appearance. This changed when a few of my patients taking collagen protein told me their hair was growing longer than they had ever been able to grow it. I knew I had to investigate further.

While there is a paucity of published studies on the effects of collagen protein on hair growth, I found a couple that pointed to possible reasons for benefits. In the first, consuming 14 grams of gelatin daily resulted in a 9 to 11 percent increase in the average diameter of individual hair strands, with some volunteers experiencing a dramatic 45 percent increase. Hair also became significantly stronger as its diameter increased. However, while the fullness of the hair increased, the length did not. And women saw greater increases in diameter than men, attributed to the fact that the men had thicker hair strands to begin with.

It could be that an overall increase in blood circulation to the scalp increases the nourishment of each hair follicle, allowing each strand to become thicker, similar effects of collagen on our fingernails. Another possibility has to do with the stem cells in our hair follicles. In experiments on mice, scientists from the University of California discovered that a special type of collagen near these stems cells, type XVII, becomes damaged with age. As this damaged collagen disappears, follicular stem cells actually turn into skin cells and slough off, causing permanent hair loss. Mice that continued to produce more of the type XVII collagen were less prone to hair loss.

These scientists then analyzed hair follicles in women ages 22 to 70, discovering that follicles in women over 55 were smaller and had lower levels of collagen XVII. Would collagen protein supplementation stop the destruction of this special type of collagen synthesized by our bodies? It might be a stretch to come to that conclusion, but it is an interesting theory.

What About Keratin Protein as a Supplement?

I wanted to be 100 percent sure that I wasn't missing anything important that could help you get the most out of your hair and nail supplementation regimen. Because keratin is incredibly resistant to digestion (heat and enzymes have almost no effect), I guessed it would have to be a special form of keratin for there to be any possibility of it being absorbed and utilized.

As a matter of fact, there is a relatively new supplement called Cynatine HNS, a form of solubilized keratin made by breaking the keratin in sheep wool into small peptides. A couple of clinical trials have been conducted and the results are interesting.

In a 2014 trial, White women between 20 and 71 years old with signs of damaged hair were given capsules containing 500 mg of solubilized keratin (Cynatine HNS), 15 mg of zinc, and 1.65 mg copper, and doses of B-vitamins, including biotin, equal to the FDA daily value. The placebo group received only capsules of maltodextrin and no supplemental vitamins or minerals. After three months, women in the Cynatine group had a 9.2 percent increase in the number of hair follicles in the growth phase and a 47 percent reduction in the number of hairs removed from the scalp after an objective "hair-pull" test by the researchers; there was no change in the placebo group. The women in the Cynatine group also had significantly greater improvements in the self-reported appearance of their hair, as well as in the hardness, smoothness, and resistance to breakage of their fingernails. Because the placebo supplement did not contain any vitamins or minerals, the possible contributions of these to the observed improvements is unknown. Zinc at that intake can definitely result in a positive impact on hair growth if someone has suboptimal zinc levels. On the other hand, the amount of biotin was nowhere near the typical daily dose efficacious in strengthening hair and nails, 5,000 to 10,000 mg.

These same researchers conducted a similar trial with the Cynatine HNS on a group of women 40 to 70 years of age who showed signs of skin aging. Those who took the Cynatine experienced a 12 percent decrease in wrinkle depth, a 17 percent improvement in skin elasticity, and a 30 percent increase in skin moisture after three months.

Should you combine collagen protein with Cynatine-brand keratin protein? That is an experiment you'll have to try on your own because to date, no studies on these taken together have been published (with the exception of anecdotal reviews, which are overwhelmingly positive). You can purchase a separate supplement containing Cynatine, or, to make it easier, there is a supplement available from Life Extension (Hair, Skin & Nails Rejuvenation Formula) that combines the tested doses of both Cynatine solubilized keratin and Verisol collagen peptides, along with a few other active ingredients. This might be worth considering for those who struggle with persistent hair or nail problems and find that collagen protein alone doesn't quite do the trick. Keep in mind that the benefits will only last if you continue to supplement with collagen or keratin or both. So whatever you choose, be prepared for a long and beautiful relationship!

CHAPTER 5

Keep Moving with Collagen

Moving through life with the fewest aches, pains, and broken bones, all while retaining strength, is a high priority for many people. Yet most of us take our skeletons, muscles, and joints for granted until something goes wrong. And when it does go wrong, our lives can be dramatically changed. I saw this firsthand when I worked in a rehabilitation center. That experience made me realize I should never take the ability to move for granted. So rather than looking at going to the gym as a chore, I try to think of it as a privilege. I hope you do, too.

If you have ever dealt with a broken bone or other physical injury, you may have thought about whether your diet has anything to do with how well your body recovers. Not every physical limitation can be overcome, but many can, to one degree or another. What you eat does make a difference. In this chapter, we'll look at the role collagen protein can play in prevention and recovery from bone loss, joint pain, muscle loss, and athletic injury.

Bones

In my practice, patients want to learn what they can do nutritionally to address a medical finding of low bone mineral density: osteopenia or osteoporosis. Osteopenia is the beginning of bone loss, and alerts doctors to monitor affected patients and recommend lifestyle changes. On the other hand, osteoporosis, diagnosed when a bone mineral density reading dips below −2.5 standard deviations from that of the average young adult, is a serious condition, more so the younger it occurs. Osteoporosis is typically treated with medications. Almost all of my patients with bone loss, either osteopenia or osteoporosis, are already taking calcium and vitamin D supplements, which can be a good start nutritionally.[3] But in order to support good bone health and prevent fractures, we need to take a wider view of what is behind this problem, which affects more than half of all people 50 years of age or older in the United States.

Bone loss is a natural part of the aging process. In women, it begins around age 30 at a rate of 0.5 percent per year, accelerates after menopause to 2 percent or more per year until about age 65, and declines steadily by 1 percent thereafter. Men in their fifties do not experience the rapid loss of bone mass that women do in the years following menopause; but by age 65, men will lose bone mass at the same rate as women. Osteoporosis is a skeletal disorder characterized not only by a significant loss of bone minerals, but also by a change in the architecture of the bone itself. You might be surprised

---

3   According to "Calcium Supplementation in Osteoporosis: Useful or Harmful?" published in *European Journal of Endocrinology*, while supplementation of calcium and vitamin D is recommended for women who have osteoporosis, calcium has not been shown to significantly reduce the risk of bone fractures and may increase risk for heart attacks.

to learn that our bones consist mostly of protein, and that 80 percent of this protein is collagen, mainly type I. And while the mineral content of our bones determines how stiff they are, the abundant collagen network actually determines their resiliency.

If you have ever had a bone mineral density test, you need to know that it only measures the amount of minerals deposited in the bone and does not reveal anything about the quality or quantity of the underlying collagen network. Because of this, not all individuals with similarly low bone mineral density can be assumed to be at equal risk. It is the age-related changes in the collagen network that reduce the mechanical strength and elasticity of bones, contributing to the occurrence of fractures. This applies to men as well, even though women are twice as likely to develop osteoporosis. A decline in estrogen decreases the maturation rate and stability of collagen, putting post-menopausal women at the highest risk. The statistics are startling: About one in every two women over 50 will break a bone because of osteoporosis.

Nothing can totally stop bone loss, but several things will help slow it down. Weight-bearing exercise, proper hormonal balance, and adequate sleep (who knew about sleep?) are three of the biggies. Nutritionally, getting sufficient vitamin D along with calcium and other minerals like magnesium and zinc is essential—it is never good to have a chronic shortfall of any of these micronutrients. Because bones are made primarily of protein, consuming adequate but not excessive protein is important as well. I find that most women are more than a little confused about what they should eat and supplement when they have osteoporosis, especially with the mixed reports on calcium that have come out recently.

How does collagen protein fit into a bone-protecting diet? Studies point to benefits for women who already have experienced bone loss, but why wait until a problem occurs? There is evidence for the bone-boosting properties of collagen protein at every age.

Throughout our youth, our bones grow longer, thicker, and stronger until peak bone mass is reached around the age of 20 for women and around the age of 30 for men. Once we are into our thirties, the best we can do is to maintain the status quo. Therefore, it is vitally important that we establish a good bone foundation while we are young. Throughout our lives, bones are in a constant state of turnover, just as is any other living tissue in our body. New bone is continuously being formed even as old bone is being broken down. But when the rate of breakdown exceeds the rate of buildup, bone loss begins to occur. In fact, most medications prescribed for osteoporosis work by interrupting the breakdown process, resulting in denser but not always better bones.[4]

How can collagen protein support the development of the bones during those very important first two to three decades of life? As you might expect, more research is needed, but collagen protein does hold promise. In the only study conducted with children, consuming hydrolyzed gelatin daily for four months resulted in positive changes in several blood markers of bone remodeling. This clinical trial, which included 60 children ages 6 to 11, indicates that daily collagen consumption appears to stimulate bone formation during critical periods of growth and development.

From studies on young rats, scientists also discovered that supplementation of hydrolyzed collagen protein promotes the development of the longest bones of the body, the femurs (thigh bones). Collagen supplementation increased not only the size and weight, but also the mineral density, stiffness, and toughness of the rat femurs. The

---

4 According to the FDA, the fracture-preventing effects of these drugs may not last beyond the few years that they are taken, but because they become part of the newly formed bone, they can stay there for years after stopping them.

scientists attributed these improvements to an increased activity of cells that synthesize bone (osteoblasts). Collagen was effective in the same doses used in humans, the equivalent of 12 grams for a 160-pound person. Since many of us will experience a broken bone sometime in our lives, it is also good to know that hydrolyzed collagen sped up the healing of femur fractures in rats. Added to the demonstrated effects on growing bone, this is good pre-clinical evidence that hydrolyzed collagen peptides hold promise in the maintenance of balanced bone turnover. It would not be an overstatement to conclude that collagen protein can help tip the scale in favor of bone formation and away from bone breakdown.

Several more studies on estrogen-deficient rats looked at the effects of collagen protein on post-menopausal bone loss. They collectively demonstrated that hydrolyzed collagen peptides can prevent bone loss by reducing inflammation and markers of bone degradation, and increasing organic bone content and markers of bone formation.

So while these findings are very intriguing, you're probably wondering what happens when real women with bone loss take collagen protein.

In the first ever clinical trial conducted on this topic, 94 post-menopausal women with clinical signs of osteoporosis were split into two groups and given either 10 grams of hydrolyzed collagen peptides or a placebo. All women were simultaneously administered twice-weekly calcitonin injections as a medical treatment for bone loss. (Calcitonin is a hormone that inhibits bone resorption when administered as a drug; it has since been replaced by newer drugs for first-line therapy). After 24 weeks, the collagen peptides enhanced the effects of calcitonin in inhibiting bone collagen breakdown as shown by a greater fall in urinary markers of bone degradation. The difference persisted three months after the treatments were discontinued. There were, however, no measurable differences in bone density between the two groups.

In a second trial, 80 seniors (with an average age of 65 years) were split into two groups: One group was given 3.5 grams of hydrolyzed collagen with glucosamine and 900 mg of algal calcium; the other received a placebo. Only the seniors in the collagen group had a decrease in a urinary marker of bone loss; they also self-reported moister and smoother skin. Two for one!

A recent study out of Florida State University used a patented type of calcium supplement, sold under the brand name KoAct. The calcium in this supplement is "chelated," or directly attached to a hydrolyzed form of type I collagen. KoAct has been effective in preventing excessive bone loss in post-menopausal women with osteopenia. In a three-month trial, the calcium-collagen chelate improved markers of bone turnover. In a separate 12-month trial, women who were given 5 grams of calcium-collagen chelate daily (supplying 500 mg of calcium and 200 IU vitamin D) experienced significantly lower levels of bone loss versus the control group (who were given 500 mg of calcium carbonate and 200 IU vitamin D). Note that the calcium-collagen chelate did not completely reverse the progression of bone loss, but it reduced the loss of bone mineral density by about two-thirds.

The consumption of collagen peptides may enhance the bioavailability of other types of dietary calcium according to one animal study. In this study, a fairly high dose of hydrolyzed collagen was used, 600 mg per kilogram of body weight of the rats, equivalent to 44 grams for a 160-pound person. But the results were remarkable—the calcium content of the rats' femurs increased by 22 percent compared to the controls, and their bone mineral density was 50 percent greater. Researchers also saw significant improvement in the bone architecture. This is about three to four times the daily amount of collagen protein thought to be safe to consume on a long-term basis, but it would be interesting to see if smaller but meaningful results could be attained with lower doses.

The most recent trial conducted with post-menopausal women was published in 2018. Conducted in Germany, the researchers divided 131 women with reduced bone mineral density into two groups. One received 5 grams daily of a specific collagen peptide, Fortibone; the other received a placebo. (At least one supplement containing Fortibone, Designs for Health Whole Body Collagen, is now available in the United States.) All of the women were encouraged to take calcium and vitamin D supplements daily. At the completion of 12 months, the collagen peptide group had an increase in the bone mineral density in the spine of almost 3 percent and a 6.7 percent increase in the femoral neck (the top of the thigh bone just below its connection to the hip, where serious fractures often occur). In the placebo group, bone density actually declined by 1.3 percent in the spine and 1 percent in the femoral neck. These results demonstrated a clear bone-building benefit of Fortibone collagen peptides, not seen previously in other clinical studies. In addition to better bones, the collagen group saw a meaningful reduction in their average blood pressure (upper and lower numbers), whereas no change occurred in the placebo group.

In one study with women diagnosed with osteopenia, the daily consumption of 10 grams of collagen peptide showed no effect on markers of bone metabolism after 24 weeks. The researchers noted that the majority of the women were overweight and therefore may have not been given a sufficient dose. They also had insufficient calcium intakes, according to an analysis of their diets, and the mean intake of vitamin B6 was about half of the Recommended Dietary Allowance. In rat studies, long-term vitamin B6 deficiency along with a higher-protein diet results in osteoporotic bone disease.

Further studies are warranted before conventional health care providers can even suggest that individuals at risk for or with active bone loss begin a collagen protein regimen. Although the chance for harm is overwhelmingly small, the cost-benefit ratio clearly remains undefined. As for my patients, I see no reason not to recommend that they supplement with collagen protein and/or gelatin along with other nutritional therapies. Even if the effects on bone are minimal, better skin, nails, and hair and more comfortable joints, as you'll see in the next chapter, are reason enough! I will touch on other bone-supportive nutritional therapies in Chapter 14. But for now, be sure not to skip over the next chapter if you have problems with joint pain or simply plan to stay active well into your advanced years.

Arthritis—Is It in Your Future?

According to the Arthritis Foundation, one in three individuals between the ages of 18 and 64 are diagnosed with arthritis or exhibit symptoms of the condition. (In this chapter, I use the word "arthritis" to refer to osteoarthritis; other forms are discussed later in the book.) The numbers get much worse after the age of 65: One in two senior men and two in three senior women will experience some degree of arthritis. Unfortunately for arthritis sufferers, there is no medical treatment without long-term side effects. Non-steroidal anti-inflammatory drugs do reduce the pain, but at a cost—prolonged use may actually inhibit the synthesis of the collagen contained in the joints. Collagen protein offers another approach that just might prevent cartilage degeneration, and in some cases may partially repair cartilage that is already damaged.

Cartilage is the type of connective tissue found in the joints, between the vertebrae, and in the airways, ears, and nose, along with a few other places in the body. Within the cartilage are chondrocytes, cells that synthesize collagen (lots of type II!), elastin, and an array of proteoglycans, all of which then get secreted into the extracellular matrix of the cartilage. The matrix of the cartilage literally soaks up water due to the presence of these special hydrophilic (water-loving) molecules called proteoglycans. Collagen gives cartilage its strength, elastin its flexibility. Because cartilage has no blood vessels to supply its chondrocytes, the nutrients these cells need arrive by way of diffusion (meaning they flow from an area of higher concentration to an area of lower concentration), making the repair of cartilage a very slow process. Movement is one way to enhance the rate of diffusion, and that is why regular exercise can be so helpful in keeping our joints healthy.

The type of collagen that covers the surfaces where two bones meet to form a joint is called articular cartilage, also referred to as hyaline cartilage, a term that comes from two Greek words meaning "transparent glass." Healthy articular/hyaline cartilage appears glassy, smooth, and well-lubricated, facilitating the movement of one bone against another with minimal friction. But when articular cartilage becomes even slightly damaged, the joints rub together like two pieces of sandpaper, causing pain that can worsen with time.

No longer accepted as an inevitability of aging, arthritis is being viewed by many baby boomers and Gen-Xers as a condition that is not only treatable, but entirely preventable. The demand for new and better non-drug therapies that do more than just reduce pain has fueled the buzz around collagen protein. Is collagen a flash in the pan or has it earned its reputation?

What Do the Studies Say?

Arthritis generally develops over a long period of time, and joints are slow to take up nutrients that can help combat it. Together, these present both opportunities and challenges in addressing arthritic changes. For true prevention, a nutritional therapy should be one that can be followed for life. And any nutritional therapy that is effective must find its way into the cartilage.

When mice were fed a diet rich in collagen hydrolysate tagged with radioactive proline, scientists observed a "pronounced and long-lasting" accumulation of the tagged hydrolysate in the cartilage of the mice. These same scientists also discovered that collagen hydrolysate stimulated lab-grown chondrocytes to synthesize greater amounts of collagen. Wanting to know how collagen hydrolysate would perform over time, these scientists then studied mice that are bred to spontaneously develop osteoarthritis. The mice's diets were supplemented with the human equivalent of 10 to 12 grams of collagen peptides daily for four months. Compared to the control mice, there was a reduction in the amount of cartilage degradation in their knees. From these pre-clinical studies, it looks like hydrolyzed collagen peptides just might help people with osteoarthritis.

In their 2012 review of the literature, researchers at the University of Rotterdam concluded that the trials to date, which included a total of six using collagen hydrolysate and two using gelatin, did not provide enough evidence to support a recommendation for collagen protein as a treatment for arthritis. A second and more rigorous review published in 2018 by researchers at the University of Sydney showed that collagen hydrolysate performed better than 17 other popular supplements[5] for improvements in pain over the short term, while scoring in the middle for medium- and longer-term improvements. I

---

5   The supplements that also scored well in this review included turmeric, boswellia, green-lipped mussel extract, glucosamine, chondroitin, avocado/soybean unsaponifiables, and vitamin D. UC-II (a special type of undenatured type II collagen) performed somewhat better than collagen hydrolysate over the longer-term, but they are thought to work very differently from each other and may quite possibly complement each other.

wanted to share this with you up front before we take a look at a few of the individual studies.

A multinational clinical study was published by a researcher from Case Western Reserve University and his colleagues, and was conducted at 20 different trial centers located across the U.S., UK, and Germany. Of almost 400 patients, half received 10 grams of a pharmaceutical-grade collagen hydrolysate, the other half a placebo, both doses taken daily for 24 weeks. Overall, in the three test countries, there was no difference between the supplement and the placebo. However, at the German site, participants receiving collagen hydrolysate experienced improvement in joint function and a reduction in pain, and the patients who had the most severe symptoms at the onset experienced the most improvement.

A trial conducted by the company Nitta Gelatin looked at the effectiveness of both porcine and bovine collagen peptides on osteoarthritis of the knee. Sixty patients, male and female, between the ages of 30 and 65 years and diagnosed with arthritis, were assigned to one of the two treatment groups; 22 others received a placebo for 14 weeks. The researchers found that the porcine collagen peptides and the bovine collagen peptides performed equally well in reducing pain and increasing joint mobility as compared to the placebo.

Chicken Collagen

Hydrolyzed collagen protein made from chicken sternal cartilage has also been tested in osteoarthritic individuals. (The sternum of a chicken is that somewhat flexible piece between the ribs that connects the two breast sections. You probably have noticed it if you have eaten chicken breasts on the bone.) Chicken sternum is rich in type II collagen, proteoglycans, and chondroitin sulfate; it closely mirrors the cartilage in human joints. This type of collagen, called hydrolyzed collagen type II,[6] is included in a wide range of supplements under the trade names BioCell and KollaGen II-xs.

To date, one study testing the effects of BioCell collagen on arthritis symptoms has been published, in the *Journal of Agricultural and Food Chemistry*. Eighty patients, all with documented progressive osteoarthritis in either their hips or knees, were divided into two groups and given either 2 grams of BioCell collagen or a placebo for 70 days. At the midpoint of the trial, the BioCell group had significant improvements in their ability to engage in physical activities. After the 10 weeks, they experienced reductions in joint pain over the placebo group. BioCell collagen also has benefits for aging skin as discussed in Chapter 4, a bonus for people suffering from arthritis.

Type II collagen from chicken sternal cartilage is also available in an "undenatured" form. Undenatured type II collagen, known simply as UC-II, is not processed with heat or enzymes and therefore is not extensively hydrolyzed like BioCell and KollaGen II-xs. According to the manufacturer (InterHealth Nutraceuticals), UC-II retains active immune modulating substances. It has been shown to help in the treatment of rheumatoid arthritis. But does it work for osteoarthritis, which is not thought to have an immune-related cause?

A clinical trial comparing the performance of UC-II to a combination of glucosamine and chondroitin (two popular over-the-counter supplements shown to have good results for reducing arthritic symptoms) was published in the *International Journal of Medical Sciences*. The blind study included 52 osteoarthritis patients ages 40 to 75, both male and female. The researchers excluded any patient with a current or past diagnosis of rheumatoid arthritis. The results showed

---

6   Hydrolyzed type II chicken collagen is different from "undenatured" type II chicken collagen or UC-II because the latter is *not* broken down into small pieces and therefore has a different mechanism of action.

that three months of daily supplementation with 40 mg of UC-II was two to three times more effective (depending on the clinical assessment utilized) than the glucosamine and chondroitin in reducing pain during daily activities.

Dog owners may want to get their best friends started on collagen protein as well. In an investigation on the effects of UC-II on dogs with moderate arthritis, three months of supplementation with this special collagen extract (4.27 grams per 1,000-calorie portion of dog food) combined with turmeric and green tea extracts resulted in a 30 percent decrease in pain, as measured by veterinary manipulation.

Benefits for Athletes Young and Old

A study out of Penn State University looked at the changes in activity-related joint pain in 147 college athletes after their daily consumption of 10 grams of collagen hydrolysate provided in a liquid form. Physicians assessed the athletes' levels of joint pain while resting, standing, walking, running, changing direction, and carrying objects. Compared to the placebo group, athletes in the collagen group experienced reduced pain during each of these activities over the 24-week study, and a subgroup of athletes with preexisting knee pain experienced an even greater reduction in pain.

To see if collagen peptides could help avert the muscle loss of aging, scientists in Germany tested them in combination with a resistance exercise program. They enrolled 53 elderly men with muscle loss in a double-blind study to see if 15 grams of collagen peptides per day (Gelita Bodybalance bovine collagen peptides) could improve muscle gains over a placebo. For 12 weeks, the men participated in a one-hour guided training program three times per week. All study participants increased their muscle mass, bone mass, and quadriceps strength, and reduced their body fat. What was interesting is that the men who were given the collagen peptides had a greater increase in muscle mass and a greater reduction in body fat. The authors of this study pointed out that other studies of comparable design, using different types of supplemental protein, did not show increases in muscle strength in elderly participants. They speculated that the high levels of glycine and arginine, which can be converted by the body into the muscle-building compound creatinine, could be one reason.

Finally, the journal *Integrative Medicine* published a very small pilot study to see whether BioCell Collagen could improve recovery from intense exercise. Eight healthy, recreationally active individuals, six men and two women, with an average age of 30 years, were split into two groups and given either 3 grams of BioCell or three grams of placebo. After six weeks of supplementation, they performed intense sets of upper-body exercises designed to result in muscle damage, then repeated these same exercises three days later. During each of the two exercise sessions, the individuals who took the BioCell had lower blood markers of muscle tissue damage and were able to perform more repetitions before failure than the placebo group.

Collagen for Mobility Issues?

I believe the evidence that collagen protein can enhance mobility and strength and reduce degenerative joint pain is just beginning to emerge. It is likely that to gain meaningful benefits, long-term consumption of collagen protein is required. I suspect that the studies have neither been long enough, nor more importantly, started early enough before significant (and often irreversible) joint damage has occurred, to give any real results.

Bottom line, don't expect quick results from collagen protein if you are suffering from arthritis. Do expect that foods and supplements rich in collagen protein and other cartilage-building nutrients will provide a wide range of benefits, including supporting healthy joints and strong muscles.

CHAPTER 6

Collagen and Your Gut Reaction

There are a number of ways that adding collagen protein and gelatin to your diet can help with digestion and overall gut health. An age-old traditional remedy has been to use homemade meat and bone broths rich in collagen protein for this purpose. In fact, entire modern-day dietary treatments revolve around the use of these broths.

Before we explore how broth-based diets work, consider today's Standard American Diet (SAD). Along with most Americans, a growing majority of the world eats the SAD. This diet is predominantly muscle meats, grains, and other cooked foods, like sandwiches, cereals, and cooked vegetables. At the same time, more and more people are adopting exclusively "raw food" diets, often with good results. Is there anything unique about raw food that can explain this popular trend?

Having dabbled in a predominantly raw food diet, I learned a few things that proponents claim about them. One, raw foods retain all their vitamins and minerals; two, they supply a lot of enzymes that help with digestion; and three, they are said to have a kind of "life force" in them. I can't agree with these statements in their entirety—some vitamins and minerals in raw foods are better retained, but others stay more locked up in the food matrix and are released by cooking; enzymes in food may or may not survive the extremely acidic environments in the stomach; and although an interesting theory, the advantage of any supposed life force in foods that we eat has little supporting data.

A key property of raw food is often overlooked: its ability to attract water as it moves through the digestive tract. This is due to the hydrophilic colloids that raw foods, especially vegetables and fruits, contain. "Hydrophilic" means water-loving, and colloids are particles that do not dissolve but become suspended in another substance. The proteins and fats in milk are a perfect example. Because of these properties, digestive juices containing stomach acid, enzymes, and bile are strongly attracted to masticated (chewed) raw foods, facilitating the multi-stage process of digestion within the gut. The longer foods are heated, the more the colloids fall out of suspension, lessening their water-attracting ability.

Unfortunately for some people, the digestion of raw foods, especially fibrous foods, can be problematic. Many of my clients do not tolerate salads and other raw vegetables well, finding they cause gas, bloating, pain, and even loose stools in some cases. Others do great on them and note they have more regular bowel movements when they eat raw fruits and vegetables daily. I believe we all have our own innate digestive capacity depending on the efficiency of our digestive organs and glands, along with the balance of bacteria in our intestines. This capacity is subject to change, as you may have experienced while recovering from a case of the stomach flu or food poisoning. The good news is that just as it can worsen, our capacity to digest can be improved as well.

How do collagen, gelatin, and bone broth play a role in improving digestion? After all, none of these are typically eaten in their raw form. The reason is that gelatin and gelatin-rich bone broths, unlike other cooked foods, form hydrophilic colloids that enhance digestion. (This is a case where hydrolyzed collagen peptides do *not* exert the same favorable effect because they lack the ability to bind to water.) Dr. Francis Pottenger Jr., a nutrition pioneer in the early part of the twentieth century, was one of the first to point out the abundance of hydrophilic colloids in broths and their great value for intestinal disorders.

Whether or not you have challenges with your digestion, I urge you to try adding bone broth or another gelatin-based food to your daily diet. You are likely to notice some remarkable benefits as the lining of your digestive tract responds. If you suffer from indigestion, colitis, or even just general bloating and discomfort, you will want to consume a cup of bone broth at least two times per day as many of my patients who find relief do. By drawing acidic digestive juices into the food, gelatin colloids both help shield the lining of the stomach and prepare the food for further digestion in the small intestine. Individuals with acid reflux may derive benefit from this protective shielding. Gelatin continues its water-attracting effects as food moves down into the colon, keeping the bowels moving more smoothly and alleviating constipation.

If making bone broth from scratch is daunting, a good alternative is adding gelatin to a store-bought broth or stock (poultry, beef, or other), around 1 tablespoon for every 1 to 2 cups. Broth can also be added to a wide variety of savory foods, replacing all or part of the water in the recipe. At the end of the book, I have included a recipe for making your own bone broth that you can use in a number of ways. Many of my patients cook their rice and quinoa in bone broth. You will also find different ways to make gelled foods like gummies and gelatin molds without all the sugar that comes with the boxed or ready-to-eat gelatin desserts.

Studies on Collagen and Digestive Health

When considering the many types of evidence that allow us to evaluate a given dietary intervention, the Academy of Nutrition and Dietetics assigns randomized controlled trials the highest grade. Clinical and anecdotal experience is ranked considerably lower in my profession's evidence-based practice model. Yet bone broth is an excellent example of the value of utilizing clinical experience. While we may not yet fully understand or appreciate its "mechanism of action" (how it actually works), we can confidently recommend bone broth based on patient results. In fact, in the early days of the dietetic profession, Dr. Pottenger noted, "[t]he use of a hydrophilic colloid in the dietetic treatment of gastric complaint is frequently sufficient in itself to rectify what are apparently serious conditions."

Collagen is the major constituent of the intestinal wall. So it would make sense that consuming collagen protein might have some effect on gastrointestinal function. Scientific studies provide clues as to just how gelatin and collagen protein work to support digestive health. Using animals and cultured cells, scientists have demonstrated the role of collagen protein in building and maintaining the connective tissue that lines the entire digestive tract. This is important because if this tissue gets damaged, it can lead to problems like leaky gut syndrome and gut inflammation. Leaky gut syndrome, known medically as increased intestinal permeability, occurs when the barrier function of the digestive tract gets disrupted, allowing undesirable molecules to pass into the body. This is discussed in greater depth in Chapter 8.

Studies done on young animals (pigs, chickens, and fish) show that consuming small quantities of the glycine and proline (0.5 to 2 percent of the diet) exerts beneficial effects on the function of the gastrointestinal tract. Glycine and proline supplementation beneficially increased the size of the intestinal villi, which are the structures that perform the final digestion and absorption of food. Additionally, these two collagen precursors increased the thickness of the intestinal mucous layer, which also plays an important role in the health and function of the digestive tract. Unsurprisingly, nutrient absorption, growth, efficiency of protein utilization, and overall collagen production were also increased. And in two separate rat studies, glycine supplementation protected the colon from the deleterious effects of radiation, while marine collagen peptides promoted the healing of stomach ulcers caused by acid erosion. These are exciting findings that suggest collagen protein may be useful for individuals suffering from damage to their digestive tract, whether due to cancer treatment, gastroesophageal reflux, celiac disease (an immune reaction to gluten), or a myriad of other causes.

Using a cellular model of the human digestive tract, scientists looked at the effects of three different sizes of marine collagen peptides on leaky gut. While the smallest peptide was the most effective, the addition of any one of the peptides prevented much of the breakdown in the tight junctions caused when a pro-inflammatory biomolecule was subsequently introduced. This emerging research points to the potential for collagen peptides to limit the increased intestinal permeability that accompanies inflammatory bowel diseases like Crohn's and underlies a host of other chronic diseases. More studies are needed, but marine collagen peptides could be a viable nutritional therapy to try in the absence of a seafood allergy.

Final Thoughts

I believe, as do other functional and integrative practitioners, that real, homemade chicken soup is not only good for the soul, it is good for the gut. It's a timeless remedy that deserves a lot more respect from the conventional medical community. Wouldn't it be great if every hospital and extended-care facility included soups made with real bone broth on the patient menu? This would probably prove to be one of the most cost-effective dietary therapies that we could offer, and one of the tastiest!

Collagen peptides also have some interesting evidence to support their use, and doubtless there will be more studies. My advice would be to go for the bone broth if your main concern is your digestive health, but make sure you prepare it with bones that have a lot of cartilage and/or skin still on them.

CHAPTER 7

Could Collagen Each Day Help Keep the Cardiologist Away?

Collagen protein has not been studied for its specific effects on cardiovascular disease in humans. There are, however, a few studies that point to a helpful role of collagen peptides on improving risk factors for heart disease and stroke, specifically in the areas of high blood pressure, dyslipidemia (such as high LDL cholesterol, high triglycerides, and low HDL cholesterol), and reduction in inflammation. And as you will learn in Chapter 9, collagen peptides are showing promise for improving blood sugar control, which could help address two of the biggest risk factors for heart disease: diabetes and prediabetes.

High Blood Pressure

High blood pressure is the most widespread risk for cardiovascular disease. But together with regular exercise and a diet rich in colorful fruits and vegetables, collagen peptides might just help people avoid the need to start on medications. Let's see what the studies say.

One small clinical trial was conducted with 15 volunteers diagnosed with mild hypertension. Their average systolic blood pressure was 136 mmHg, 16 points higher than the recommended upper number. All 15 volunteers were given 5.2 grams of a chicken collagen hydrolysate containing a unique "octapeptide," meaning it was eight amino acids in length. After four weeks of daily consumption, the average systolic blood pressure dropped by nearly 12 points. The chicken collagen worked in a similar way to high blood pressure medications, but without the side effects seen with commonly prescribed ACE inhibitors, such as dry cough. In their commentary, the authors mentioned the time-honored use of chicken soup as part of *yakuzen* (herbal medicine–based Chinese foods) for improvement of poor blood circulation. It appears that traditional medicine is onto something!

In a larger placebo-controlled trial with 58 volunteers, the same Japanese scientists again tested chicken collagen hydrolysate, this time against a placebo. Thirty men and 28 women with either mild hypertension or high-normal blood pressure who were not taking blood pressure medications were included. They were randomly assigned to receive either 2.9 grams of chicken collagen hydrolysate mixed into a fermented beverage or the identical beverage without the collagen. After 12 weeks of daily consumption, the collagen group's average systolic blood pressure dropped from 141.1 to 131.8, while the average systolic pressure of the placebo group did not change. As expected, the blood pressure–lowering effects ended after stopping the chicken collagen–containing beverage.

Both of these studies used specially prepared chicken collagen hydrolysates, so other types of collagen protein may or may not produce equivalent results. However, bovine collagen may also have a degree of blood pressure–lowering properties.

In a clinical trial designed to measure the effects of a specific bovine collagen peptide (Fortibone) on bone retention in post-menopausal women diagnosed with osteopenia, researchers noted a statistically significant blood pressure–lowering effect. At the end of 12 months, 5 grams of Fortibone per day lowered average systolic (128.1 versus 134.5 mmHg) and diastolic (78.6 versus 81.2 mmHg) blood pressures as compared to the placebo group, whose blood pressure did not change. Although not something the researchers set out to measure, these small reductions in blood pressure were a nice side effect of the collagen protein.

While we wait for more human trials, the results from animal studies point to blood pressure–normalizing benefits in other types of collagen peptides. In studies on rats, chicken collagen hydrolysate produced blood pressure–lowering effects. Perhaps even more interesting was the collagen's ability to increase nitric oxide concentration and reduce damage to the cardiovascular system. Nitric oxide relaxes the blood vessels, allowing them to dilate, boosting blood flow, and helping to lower blood pressure.

Also seen in rat studies, bovine and porcine collagen peptides have blood pressure–lowering activity nearly 40 percent as effective as ACE-inhibiting medications; these collagen peptides are currently available to the consumer. The most active forms of collagen peptides studied have been pre-filtered to concentrate their active ingredients. In addition to the existing products on the market, these and other targeted types of collagen peptides may become available to consumers sometime in the future. Until then, homemade chicken broth could just be the ticket.

Cholesterol and Other Risk Factors for Heart Disease

There is little research on whether collagen protein has any effect on blood cholesterol and other risk factors for heart disease. The only clinical study to date testing the effect of collagen protein on cholesterol was conducted in China with 100 patients who had type 2 diabetes. These patients were randomly divided into two groups, one given 13 grams of marine collagen peptides daily, the other a placebo, for three months. Not only were their blood levels of triglycerides, LDL cholesterol, and fasting blood sugar significantly lower, but the collagen peptides also reduced overall inflammation, increased HDL (good) cholesterol, and improved insulin sensitivity.

When scientists fed rats diets containing 0.17 percent fish collagen peptides, they observed a lowering of total blood lipids and triglycerides. And in a separate experiment, the same scientists discovered that the addition of fish collagen peptides to a one-time feeding of soybean oil lowered the rats' triglycerides two hours later.

Inflammation is now understood to be a risk factor behind many chronic diseases, including heart disease. It is too early to conclude that collagen protein can reduce inflammation within the arterial wall, a chronic type of inflammation that underlies the development of coronary artery disease. In animal studies, collagen peptides not only lowered bad cholesterol, they also reduced markers of inflammation. Specifically, mice fed a diet with 10 percent chicken collagen hydrolysate for 12 weeks had significantly lower concentrations of several pro-inflammatory molecules in their blood than mice on a standard diet. They also had less accumulation of fat in their livers. Fatty liver disease is another widespread risk factor for heart disease and is strongly associated with undesirable changes in blood lipids, higher risk for diabetes, and higher coronary calcium scores (a test measuring blockage of the coronary arteries).

What great news that while you are beautifying the appearance of your outer self with collagen protein, especially from chicken, you could very well be protecting the health of your inner self! I am more convinced now than ever that we all need to eat more chicken soup. And to help you do just that, I have included a few recipes that will make eating chicken broth anything but boring (page 169).

CHAPTER 8

Weighing In on Collagen

Are you searching for the perfect diet plan that will end your struggles with weight forever? Perhaps you have never been overweight but are experiencing undesirable shifts in body fat that set in with age, coinciding with a loss of muscle. Could collagen protein help you build and maintain a better body composition?

Weight Loss

To be clear, no single food or supplement is a magic bullet: No special protein, fat, vegetable, fruit, or herb will lead to weight loss all on its own. A moderately lower-calorie diet that is nutritionally complete and manages cravings and hunger is the only dietary prescription for weight loss that I have seen to work. When trying but not succeeding in losing weight, I find there are three major things the majority of my patients have done wrong in the past: One, attempting to lose weight too rapidly; two, meal patterns that fall short on one or more micronutrients; and three, trying to do it all with diet alone, while not fixing poor sleep, stress, and exercise habits.

MACRONUTRIENT RATIOS FOR WEIGHT LOSS

Wondering what macronutrient ratios I recommend for weight loss? It depends on the client, but I generally recommend a low carb, moderate fat diet, with sufficient but not excessive protein. I rarely recommend ketogenic diets unless a patient has been referred to me by a physician who prescribes this, or the patient desires to give this a try. Ketogenic diets often do work, at least in the short term, but I have seen weights plateau on these diets when followed for more than a few months. For women especially, a lowering of metabolic rate is not unusual, leading to a lifetime of restricting food to maintain the desired weight.

To lose weight and keep it off, slower is often better than faster. A slower pace, around 2 to 4 pounds per month, can minimize the degree to which the body's "famine survival" mechanism kicks in. Simply put, the more weight that is lost, the more the body wants to hold on to its remaining fat stores and then work to replace them once the dieting ends. This is due in part to a lowering of the body's metabolic rate, which is responsible for the plateau that dieters often hit after initial weight-loss success. As of now, there are no studies to show collagen protein can prevent a plateauing of weight, but this is still important to know so you can avoid one of the most common pitfalls dieters face.

After educating my patients on the need to be tortoises instead of hares on their way to the weight-loss finish line, we work to eliminate the other problems standing in their way. Stress, lack of sleep, under-and overexercising, hormonal imbalances, toxic burdens, and poor gut health are some of the main contributors to weight gain outside of excess calories. A big problem that I see is micronutrient deficiencies, often made worse by years of dieting. Once we begin to address all of these concerns and make sure the patient is eating real, nourishing foods, their overall health improves and they start to see weight come off and stay off.

How does collagen protein fit into your personal nutrition prescription for weight management? Here is where bone broth and gelatin, along with collagen peptides, would be the dietary treatment of choice.

Leaky Gut and Metabolic Distress

Increasingly recognized as a pervasive health problem, intestinal permeability, a.k.a. "leaky gut," could very well be underlying many people's weight problems, along with many other chronic diseases.

Our gastrointestinal tract (GI tract, for short) and specifically our intestines are lined with food-digesting cells which pack together to form "tight junctions" that prevent undigested food particles from slipping between them. This keeps the contents of our GI tract isolated from our bloodstream until the entire digestive process is completed. But when our GI tract is exposed to inflammatory foods, pathogenic bacteria, environmental toxins, and many types of medications, not to mention too much alcohol, too much stress, and too little sleep, gaps in these tight junctions can occur.

When this happens, undigested food particles find their way through these gaps into the bloodstream, along with bacterial toxins and other undesirables. As these foreign invaders are identified and targeted by the immune system, an immune response triggers an increase in system-wide inflammation. If the inflammation continues unabated, what often occurs is a gradual increase in body fat or an inability to lose existing body fat, problems compounded by a gradual decline in muscle mass.

As mentioned in Chapter 6, there are dietary protocols that focus on healing and sealing a severely leaky gut. The foundational food in these protocols is homemade broth made with cartilaginous and skin-covered bones. Although there is a medical test that can detect the presence of leaky gut, I've rarely seen it ordered by a conventional doctor. My educated guess is that almost everyone has a degree of leakiness in their guts, depending on the degree of unhealthy lifestyle factors mentioned previously. I consider this a problem that needs to be addressed in almost every overweight patient, and advise them to consume bone broths (homemade or purchased and prepared with added gelatin) at least twice per day. This is not the entire protocol, of course, but it is often where we begin. Patients who follow this recommendation are often surprised that their hunger diminishes, their bowel movements are more regular, and even their mental clarity increases. Over time, their weight slowly comes down, especially when they work to address all other concerns.

Does published evidence support this clinical experience with patients? Not exactly, but there is a growing body of evidence demonstrating the associations between leaky gut and metabolic diseases such as obesity, diabetes, and fatty liver disease. In addition, patients with these metabolic problems show higher levels of bacterial toxins in their bloodstream. Probiotics and probiotic-rich foods, especially when added to a balanced diet rich in gelatin or bone broth, will further protect the integrity of the intestinal lining.

Collagen, Hunger, and Fullness

Studies have shown that when people include more protein in their diet, they reduce their food intake, lose weight, and better maintain weight loss after dieting. Meals containing adequate amounts of protein (20 to 40 grams, or about 3 to 6 ounces) suppress hunger more effectively and longer than do lower-protein meals. Knowing which types of protein satiate best is key, because almost every dieter will eventually be sabotaged by hunger, which tends to increase as more weight is lost. One of the reasons the popular low-carb ketogenic diet is so effective is that hunger is often less of a problem, in part because more protein is being consumed, but also because blood sugar levels become stabilized. When hunger is less, individuals find it easier to consume fewer calories. However, a "keto" diet is not right for everyone and may not be right for you. Still, you need effective ways to keep hunger at bay.

As you might expect, when looking at how well various proteins satiate hunger, there are differences. Types of collagen protein, specifically gelatin and hydrolyzed gelatin, have been put to the test for their effects on hunger and hormones that control sensations of hunger. Let's see how they stack up.

A single-day study was conducted with 24 healthy adult volunteers. For breakfast, they were given a custard made from one of seven different types of protein. Two of the proteins, gelatin and alpha-lactalbumin (derived from dairy), were found to be 40 percent more satiating than the others, which included whey, casein, and soy protein. At lunch, three hours later, the volunteers who had eaten the custards containing the gelatin or alpha-lactalbumin consumed 20 percent fewer calories, even though they were offered the same foods the control group received. A subsequent experiment by the same research team showed that alpha-lactalbumin protein was better at suppressing appetite four hours after consumption, compared with gelatin.

Another study by the same research group looked at diets containing either gelatin or casein as the sole source of protein and measured differences in appetite suppression, protein utilization, and rates of energy expenditure. In this short-term study with 23 healthy men and women, gelatin suppressed hunger 44 percent more than the casein but caused the participants to lose a small amount of body protein, while casein preserved their protein stores better. The amount of energy expended by the participants did not differ between the two proteins. Because gelatin is not a complete protein, the loss of body protein was not unexpected. The researchers concluded that the addition of gelatin and casein to a weight-loss diet could both suppress hunger and preserve muscle and bone mass.

My suggestion here is to add collagen protein, whether in the form of broth, gelatin, or peptides, to your breakfast and see if you notice a reduction in your hunger before lunchtime. Two scrambled eggs with cheese (casein) or yogurt (casein and whey) and a fruited gelatin is one option. A bowl of homemade soup with 3 ounces of chicken is perfect for those who like to break out from the routine. If you prefer a portable breakfast, try a smoothie made using 10 grams of collagen protein and 20 grams of whey protein (20 percent alpha-lactalbumin). Experiment to see which meals work for you; all should supply at least 25 grams of protein and 400 to 600 calories for best results. In Chapter 10, I'll discuss another important reason why you will want to combine whey protein with your collagen protein.

In a third single-day study by the same researchers, 12 obese and 10 normal-weight volunteers were given a flavored, sweetened gelatin (20 grams by dry weight) to eat. Afterward, their blood was drawn every 30 minutes over a three-hour period to measure the levels of several hormones that control hunger and satiety. The single-gelatin meal raised both insulin and GLP-1 (a hormone that helps promote insulin secretion and replenishes the pancreatic stores of insulin), which the researchers suggested would help maximize satiety and thus improve adherence to lower-calorie diets.

Animal Studies on Collagen for Weight Management

I think researchers will continue to study how collagen and gelatin proteins can play beneficial roles in weight management. It would be fantastic if collagen protein proved to be a magic bullet, but even as more studies come out, that appears extremely unlikely. Yet studies done on rats give additional reason to feel good about collagen protein as a weight-management tool.

Scientists wanted to find out if hydrolyzed collagen might offer any help for the problem of menopausal weight gain. They removed the ovaries from rats—to mimic the low estrogen levels that follow menopause in women—and then studied the effects of two different concentrations of collagen protein supplied in the rats' drinking water. The higher concentration of collagen protein, 2.5 mg/ml (equivalent to 5 grams in 2 liters of water), significantly slowed the rate of weight gain and the enlargement of fat cells in the rats. The scientists concluded, "collagen supplementation is beneficial for menopause-induced obesity."

Post-menopause is a time when women put on more fat around their midsection. Unfortunately, this happens even to women who have always eaten a healthy diet and maintained an ideal body weight. Many of my female patients meet with me specifically to address this unwelcome change in their shape; they want to lose their "menopot." What they don't always know is that this abdominal weight gain predisposes them to a higher risk for prediabetes and cardiovascular disease.[7]

One of the contributors to abdominal weight or "belly fat" are diets higher in refined carbohydrates, especially sugar. To understand the effects of supplemental glycine on diets high in sugar, in the second study a team of scientists added 30 percent sugar to the drinking water of healthy male rats. (The extra calories from the sugar was offset by a spontaneous and equivalent reduction in calories from their regular food.) After four weeks, they then added glycine (1 percent concentration) to the sugar water of one group of rats, while the control group continued to drink pure sugar water. The scientists found that the addition of glycine to the rats' sugar water significantly reduced their levels of abdominal fat, triglycerides, and insulin. The results were comparable to those measured in rats who had always drank just plain water (no sugar and no glycine). This points to a protective effect of collagen protein, rich in glycine, against the accumulation of belly fat. It may be possible with collagen protein to "have your (small slice of) cake and eat it too!"

Collagen and Weight-Loss "Shrink"

When a person has a lot of weight to lose, a concern is how to limit excessive skin hanging down from where the underlying fat has shrunk. Unfortunately, the skin can only be stretched so far and for so long before it loses some of its elasticity. As you read in Chapter 4, collagen protein helps skin become more elastic, enabling it to stretch and bounce back more readily. It may be a long time before

---

7   According to "The Role of Weight in Postmenopausal Women's Longevity" in *ScienceDaily*, being overweight after menopause is not associated with all-cause mortality in women unless it is accompanied by a higher waist circumference.

we see a study on the effects of collagen protein on skin tautness during and following weight loss. My recommendation for anyone with any amount of weight to lose is to do it slowly, eat a diet rich in protein, and include bone broth, gelatin, and collagen peptides for all the reasons mentioned here. As a bonus, collagen proteins might just help tighten loose skin.

CHAPTER 9

Collagen: The Right Protein for Optimizing Blood Sugar

When I first started in private practice a decade ago, it was rare that patients brought in bloodwork that included a hemoglobin A1c level unless they had a diagnosis of diabetes. Known simply as HbA1c, or even "A1c," this blood marker provides an estimate of two to three months of blood sugar levels, with normal being less than or equal to 5.6 percent and optimal closer to 5.0. Nowadays, an A1c test has become fairly routine for patients who are overweight, older, have high fasting blood glucose levels, high blood pressure, high blood lipids, polycystic ovary syndrome, a history of gestational diabetes, or a combination of any or all of these risk factors. Because even a slightly elevated A1c level can signal that a person is heading for diabetes unless significant lifestyle changes are made, I recommend that almost everyone get an A1c check periodically.

"Prediabetes is diabetes," according to Dr. Leigh Perreault from the University of Colorado Anschutz Medical School. This may seem like an overstatement, but the truth is that unless preemptive steps are taken, 70 percent of people with prediabetes, diagnosed when fasting blood glucose is between 100 and 125, will go on to develop diabetes. The good news is that individuals with prediabetes who get their blood glucose back into the normal range are less than half as likely to go on to develop full diabetes.

For a patient diagnosed with diabetes, the first dietary changes nutritionists recommend should include a reduction in the overall intake of carbohydrates. This will reduce elevated blood glucose and A1c in almost every case. However, it is doubtful that the worldwide diabetes epidemic, affecting 425 million people and forecasted to affect 592 million, or 1 in 10 adults by 2035, is driven simply by a surplus of carbohydrates in the diet. I share a broader view with other nutrition experts that the risk factors contributing to diabetes are both numerous and complex. This viewpoint, which has been gaining more attention, attributes diabetes to problems that inevitably develop when we live far removed from an ancestral diet and lifestyle. These problems are compounded by the plethora of endocrine-disrupting chemicals, electromagnetic fields, and light pollution in our modern environment. All are suspected to contribute to deleterious metabolic changes that can begin before a person is even born.

Unfortunately, undoing all of the adverse metabolic changes is not always possible. Yet each step taken builds upon the others, empowering an individual to live a long, healthy, and productive life despite underlying insulin resistance and a history of blood sugar problems. In addition to reducing the intake of carbohydrates, another positive dietary step is to moderately increase the intake of protein. Compared to carbohydrate, protein ingestion results in little or no increase in blood glucose levels. Protein also stimulates the release of the two main hormones that regulate blood glucose: insulin and glucagon, the blood sugar–raising hormone. Collagen protein may be even more effective than other proteins in regulating blood glucose.

Let me emphasize that supplementing a balanced diet with collagen protein is not a medical treatment for diabetes. Treating any disease, including diabetes, is beyond the scope of this book. At the same time, there are intriguing studies that show benefits to including collagen protein and gelatin in the diet. Even as early as the 1900s, a published medical report indicated that gelatin was being used successfully in the treatment of diabetes. This practice has modern-day evidence behind it—some of the reasons are the high levels of glycine in gelatin and in collagen protein. But there is more to collagen protein than just the effects of glycine. Scientists have been looking into the ways hydrolyzed collagen protein can improve blood sugar control and reduce the risk for the health problems that accompany prediabetes and diabetes. The published studies largely come out of Japan and China using targeted types of marine collagen peptides. While there are only a couple of clinical trials as of now, the results are promising.

In a study with 100 Chinese patients with type 2 diabetes randomly split into two groups, one group received 13 grams of fish collagen peptides daily, the second a placebo. By the midpoint of this three-month clinical trial, the patients consuming the collagen peptides had significant reductions in fasting blood glucose and HbA1c; their serum lipid profile improved, evidenced by lower triglycerides and LDL cholesterol and higher HDL cholesterol; and they had a decrease in markers of inflammation. These improvements were sustained through the duration of the trial.

In a related report, again on the effects of daily consumption of 13 grams of fish collagen peptides, this same group of Chinese patients with diabetes had beneficial decreases in blood levels of free-circulating fatty acids and markers of metabolic dysregulation and inflammation, and beneficial increases in hormones that support healthy glucose and blood pressure levels. The researchers suggested their findings pointed to a protective effect at the nuclear receptor level (the "control center" of all cells), one that could potentially slow the progression of diabetes and high blood pressure. They proposed that further study could lead to the development of diabetes drugs based on marine collagen peptides.

Research using cell and animal models suggests another way in which marine collagen peptides may lessen the impact of diabetes. From these studies, scientists discovered that hydrolyzed collagen effectively inhibits the enzyme dipeptidyl-peptidase IV, working much in the same way that blood sugar–lowering drugs known as DPP-4 inhibitors do. Intended for people who need more intensive medical management, DPP-4 inhibitors are a newer class of drugs that, while effective, now carry an FDA warning because some patients have developed severe joint pain while taking them. As we wait for more clinical trials to be done on collagen protein, the good news is it just might play a role in a healthy blood sugar–lowering diet while alleviating joint pain, a potential alternative to the traditionally prescribed medications.

The Case for Eating Meat

Protein in higher amounts is helpful, but isn't meat something to avoid?

In my practice I utilize a food frequency checklist to see how often patients eat from various categories of foods. In the red meat category, the vast majority of patients indicate fewer than three times per week, with many reporting zero times per week. When I ask their reasons for an infrequent intake (although I pretty much know the answer before I ask) the typical response is, "I've been trying to avoid red meat." Does that describe you as well?

Red meat—unless you're a paleo or low-carb diet adherent, the idea of eating it does not align with what you might consider healthy dietary practices. Epidemiological studies have associated red meat with almost every chronic disease known to humans: diabetes, cancer, heart disease, and even a shortened lifespan. Does it deserve this reputation? Maybe, but then again maybe not. It depends. That may sound like I am dodging the question, but the truth is we cannot look at any single food in isolation, and we should avoid making one-size-fits-all dietary recommendations.

There are legitimate concerns that put red meat in the headlines, including the following: Red meats are often eaten grilled or preserved with nitrates, and both methods of preparation imbue the meat with some degree of carcinogens; red meat is rich in iron, which for some people can detrimentally accumulate in the body; red-meat eaters may not consume enough plant-based foods to balance their meat intake; and red meat is rich in the essential amino acid methionine, which is thought to be harmful in excess, especially when the diet is low in glycine. If this last reason is news to you, you're not alone. Many nutritionists don't know anything about it either. But this reason is important, and it tells us why collagen protein is especially important for meat eaters.

Glycine Is a Superhero

In Chapter 3, I introduced glycine, the little amino acid that can. Studies show that most people do not consume enough of this conditionally essential amino acid. To make matters worse, low intakes of glycine along with high intakes of methionine are particularly harmful.[8] This was first observed in rodent studies: Rats on high-methionine diets had shorter lifespans than those on low-methionine diets. A subsequent experiment discovered that when glycine was added to a high-methionine diet, rats lived significantly longer and had lower glucose and triglyceride levels. These findings underscore the wisdom of traditional diets that balanced "muscle" meats rich in methionine with "gelatinous" meats (connected to the bone or covered with skin) rich in glycine. Collagen protein offers a potential strategy for living longer and stronger—so you won't have to give up the benefits of higher protein that can forestall muscle and bone loss in the context of a diet containing a good balance of plant foods.

How do these findings relate to blood sugar control and the risk for diabetes in humans? In a study of almost 28,000 individuals, researchers found that the highest intake of red meat was associated with a 25 percent increased risk for type 2 diabetes, an association that disappeared with high intakes of glycine, along with low ferritin levels (a storage form of iron) and low levels of liver-derived circulating fats.

People with type 2 diabetes, prediabetes, and obesity have been shown to have lower levels of glycine in their blood. The state of insulin resistance that accompanies these conditions leads to a metabolic loss of glycine. Some researchers have proposed that reduced glycine levels can be a reliable predictor of diabetes as early as seven years before a diagnosis is made. These lower levels actually improve with weight loss, regular exercise, and certain insulin-sensitizing medications, indicating that the amount of glycine in the blood does not solely reflect dietary intake.

---

8 Methionine restriction is a focus of research on lifespan extension in humans. In 2014, an international group of scientists convened in Tarrytown, New York, to share emerging research on this topic. Read "The First International Mini-Symposium on Methionine Restriction and Lifespan" in *Frontiers in Genetics* for more.

DON'T FORGET ABOUT PROLINE

Do these results indicate that collagen and gelatin could be helpful for managing blood sugar simply because of the high glycine content? Before you go out and buy glycine supplements, consider a second study where the same researchers from the previous study looked at proline's effect on blood glucose. They found that consuming the amino acid proline together with the same 25 grams of glucose blunted the overall rise in blood glucose by almost one-quarter as compared to glucose alone, with no change in insulin output. Not quite the solo performance of glycine, but this dynamic duo is easily obtained by consuming collagen protein, which is 23 percent proline/hydroxyproline and 33 percent glycine.

What is even more interesting about glycine is that it appears to blunt the rise in blood glucose that typically follows a high-carbohydrate meal or snack. A study done with nine healthy individuals showed that consuming about 4.5 grams of glycine along with 25 grams of glucose (roughly the same amount in three-quarters cup of mashed potato) reduced the overall increase in blood glucose to just half of that observed when the amount of glucose was consumed alone. Additionally, the glycine caused their glucose to return to fasting levels more quickly. These are two things that, over time, could help to lower an elevated HbA1c—definitely what people with diabetes want to see!

In this study, only a modest increase in insulin output occurred when glycine and glucose were consumed together, so higher insulin levels did not fully explain the remarkable decrease in blood glucose. The researchers hypothesized that the lower glucose response was in part due to glycine stimulating the release of a gut hormone that helps insulin to work better. (One of insulin's main roles is to move glucose from the bloodstream into the various cells in our bodies.) What was also interesting was that when consumed alone (without glucose), glycine stimulated an increase in glucagon, the major hormone responsible for raising blood sugar during fasting. Although small, this study does suggest that collagen protein, rich in glycine, may act to keep blood sugar on a more even keel. Blunting the highs and lows of blood sugar is something that everyone can benefit from, diabetes or not.

Low Blood Sugar and Collagen Protein

Perhaps you have experienced the symptoms of reactive hypoglycemia, or a rapid drop in blood sugar levels that occurs within four hours after eating. If so, you know how life-altering this condition can be, causing extreme hunger, unusual fatigue, brain fog, mood changes, and in the worst cases, nausea, sweating, shakiness, and lightheadedness. When it occurs in the middle of the night, you may wake with a start and then have difficulty getting back to sleep.

Did you know that the symptoms of low blood sugar can signal that your body may be on the path to insulin resistance? Insulin resistance happens when the body's cells stop fully responding to the insulin signal your pancreas is sending out. As a result, the brain instructs your pancreas to "shout louder" and release more insulin. Those high insulin levels could very well be behind the sudden drops in blood sugar. And if insulin resistance goes on unabated, it poses a high risk for progressing to prediabetes and eventually even diabetes. Many people who have hypoglycemia are not overweight, so they never suspect they could be at risk for insulin resistance, much less diabetes.

The human body has elaborate regulatory mechanisms that work to keep blood sugar, or blood glucose, in a relatively narrow range. Insulin and glucagon are the two main hormones that regulate this process and their actions "oppose" each other: Insulin lowers blood glucose, whereas glucagon raises it. Your body continually manages the release of both of these from your pancreas, and when it's working right, you aren't even aware of the ongoing adjustments. It is when they are out of sync, so to speak, with insulin predominating over glucagon, that the problem of low blood sugar can arise.

Many patients with symptoms of low blood sugar simply believe that this is their "normal." They tell me their routine is to eat every two to three hours, which keeps their "hunger" problem under control. While a protein and carbohydrate snack does alleviate the symptoms in the short term, my goal is to prevent them from experiencing a sudden drop in blood sugar in the first place. Several things contribute to reactive hypoglycemia, and we work systematically to address the issues surrounding diet, sleep, and stress. I often determine that they are actually undernourished and then work to rectify inadequate protein, fat, magnesium, zinc, and vitamin B6 intakes, along with other micronutrient shortfalls.

I recently added a few new tools to my box for patients with hypoglycemia: collagen protein, gelatin, and bone broth. Regular consumption of these can help for several reasons: One, glycine and proline are among the amino acids that can be converted to glucose as the body requires; two, glycine has been shown in cell studies to stimulate the release of glucagon from the pancreas; and three, lycine and proline lower peak glucose levels in human subjects who consume them simultaneously with glucose. When glucose levels descend rapidly, the brain senses that there is a potentially life-threatening situation occurring. The body reacts by releasing adrenaline, which raises blood glucose but also causes agitation and shakiness.

Try adding some collagen protein, gelatin, or bone broth to each balanced meal and see what happens. As your blood sugar peaks and valleys begin to level out, symptoms begin to go away. You just might find that you don't need to snack anywhere near as often and that your midafternoon caffeine boost isn't quite as necessary. Just make sure you address other potential causes of hypoglycemia, because collagen protein cannot do the work all by itself.

Whether or not you think you are currently dealing with blood sugar issues, don't be surprised if you experience more energy and clearer thinking, along with better numbers on your next blood work, after introducing collagen protein to you diet.

Amino Acids and Collagen

Collagen protein is rich in three special amino acids—glycine, and proline and hydroxyproline (which later converts to proline)—which make up more than half of collagen.

The Role of Glycine

Let's start with glycine, because it has some of the most significant roles to play in the body, yet sadly is often in short supply in our diets, as you learned in Chapter 3.

Cancer

The connection between glycine and cancer deserves more attention, especially considering the increase in cancer rates and the low amounts of glycine in the modern diet. The available studies suggest collagen protein and gelatin have a protective effect due to their high content of glycine, but this by no means allows us to conclude that collagen is a proven cure for cancer. However, because there is virtually no harm in consuming a moderate amount of collagen or gelatin on a daily basis, you can feel good that by doing so, you may be improving your odds against cancer. Let's look at what the data from animal studies suggests.

Two separate experiments were conducted by scientists from the University of North Carolina, both measuring the effects of glycine on experimentally induced melanoma in mice. In the first, they substituted glycine for one quarter of the protein content in the diet of the experimental group of mice. After two weeks, they compared the growth of the tumors in the mice fed glycine to that of the mice on the control diet. The glycine inhibited the growth of melanoma by more than 50 percent and resulted in 70 percent fewer blood vessels supplying these tumors as they formed.

In a second experiment, they studied the effects of a diet containing 5 percent glycine, versus a control diet, on the growth of experimentally induced liver cancer. At the end of one year, the glycine-supplemented mice had a 23 percent reduction in the number of small liver tumors and a 64 percent reduction in the size of medium tumors.

Another team of scientists in Tokyo and at the University of North Carolina discovered that glycine interferes with the development of new blood vessels that fuel cancer cells, a process known as angiogenesis, to inhibit the growth of tumors. They proposed that glycine could be used as a treatment to reduce inflammation as well as to prevent and treat cancer. Chronic inflammation is considered to be a factor that can increase the risk for cancer. Additional experiments on animals have confirmed that glycine is both an anti-inflammatory and immune-supporting nutrient.

To date, only one study has tested the effects of collagen protein on cancer. Chinese scientists found that marine collagen peptides increased the lifespan and decreased the incidence of spontaneous malignant tumors in rats. In this experiment, rats were fed diets supplemented with varying amounts of collagen peptides (0 to 9 percent by weight) and observed until their natural death. No cancer-inducing chemical was introduced. The collagen peptides were effective at dietary concentrations of 4.5 percent for the male rats and 9 percent for the female rats. There was no difference in food intake or body weight between the test rats and the controls, which did not receive collagen peptides. This is important because most rodent studies that demonstrate life-extending properties of a tested supplement fail to report on food intake, making it unclear if an increase in longevity could be due to caloric restriction.

On the other hand, could collagen protein have cancer-promoting effects? In 2017, scientists from the UK demonstrated that a diet completely devoid of glycine and serine slowed down the growth of lymphoma and intestinal cancer in mice. This latest study would suggest that for some people diagnosed with cancer, consuming glycine-rich collagen protein is not such a good idea. Could one of the foods traditionally considered healing and fortifying, homemade chicken soup, actually be harmful to cancer patients? Seeking the best advice, I looked for additional research on the glycine–cancer connection. What I found was that according to two studies done in cancer cell lines, glycine increased rates of cancer growth. In breast cancer patients, a higher activity of genes involved in glycine metabolism was associated with higher mortality.

I discovered a detailed explanation from Joel Brind, professor of biology and endocrinology at Baruch College and a medical research biochemist since 1981. His explanation is somewhat scientific, but it made a lot of sense to me: "[These two studies] offer hard evidence that many human cancers are selected for, and therefore arise in, bodies which are chronically methionine-loaded and glycine-deficient. Thus, they underscore the need for the proper balance between glycine and methionine." However, Dr. Brind added that during chemotherapy, "glycine supplementation may be counterproductive."

Mental Health

Glycine plays an intriguing role in the stability of our mood and overall mental state. It works in partnership with the essential amino acid methionine. Methionine is a fundamental nutrient needed for the process of methylation, which, among other very important functions, regulates the neurotransmitter dopamine. To greatly simplify, we need to methylate (or add a carbon molecule to) dopamine in the right proportion in order to maintain a balance between mental stability and mental flexibility. Too little methylation and we tend to get "stuck" on thoughts; too much, and we may behave in unpredictable and abrupt ways.

Many factors determine how we methylate, genetics playing the largest role. Nutritionists tend to think of vitamins like folate and B12 as key supporting players, but an often overlooked factor is the amount of protein, and especially animal protein, in our diets. If we eat an omnivorous diet that is largely based on methionine-rich animal protein, we may risk an undesirable increase in dopamine methylation.

Here is where glycine is helpful. When we eat foods rich in both glycine and methionine (for example, chicken or fish with the skin and meat cooked on the bone), the glycine prevents the excessive methylation of dopamine, which is exactly what we want. In effect, this balanced way of eating keeps our brains on a more even keel.

Since animal proteins are much higher in methionine than plant proteins are, strict vegetarians take in about one-quarter the amount of methionine, substantially decreasing the raw material needed for methylation. Due to this, vegetarians tend to be more at risk for under-methylation than overmethylation. On the other hand, vegetarians are also likely to have low levels of glycine in their diets, exhibiting almost double the levels of a urinary marker for glycine deficiency than omnivores. And even omnivores have substantial amounts of the urinary marker for glycine deficiency, probably because they typically fail to include skin and bone in their diets.

Ideally, our diets should provide a balance of both methionine and glycine to optimize our genetically programmed mental traits. Since the skin is three times richer in glycine than the meat, and the bones are six times richer in glycine than meat, the nutrition prescription for optimizing mental health is the same one we need for optimizing physical health: Eat skin and bones (or broth made from these) along with meat, and if not, add collagen protein to your diet.

Sleep

Good mental health depends on a complex interplay of physical, psychological, and sociological factors. We need to eat well, be physically active, know and express our life purpose, enjoy pleasurable activities, have meaningful relationships, and rest when we are tired. Not an easy list to fulfill, and there is often little time for rest and relaxation. Since I work with a lot of women in their forties, fifties, and sixties, I am acutely attuned to the chronic sleep disruption that can arise when a woman's metaphorical plate becomes overloaded and her hormones begin to change.

To address sleep issues, the first place I start is with a de-stress protocol. Although many people do not realize it, dieting can be very stressful to our well-being, especially when combined with frequently skipping meals. Undereating, overexercising, low levels of pleasurable activities, and long to-do lists that never seem to shrink further pile on to the stress load. Now compound this with extended screen time without seeing the literal light of day, and you have the ideal recipe for circadian rhythm disruption—or how to confuse your body so that it doesn't know when to be awake and when to be asleep.

While we work on all the major lifestyle contributors to poor sleep, many patients ask me what they can take to relax and fall asleep more easily, without making them drowsy the following day. While a number of herbs can be helpful, that is not my first go-to. I often suggest that they begin with a trial of glycine, 3 grams taken right before bedtime. This same remedy was tested in a group of eight female and three male volunteers who had been continuously experiencing unsatisfactory sleep. In this trial over 2 consecutive nights, 3 grams of glycine at bedtime was shown to improve both the quantity and quality of sleep, shortening the time to fall asleep without interfering with normal sleep architecture. The volunteers also reported reduced daytime sleepiness and exhibited better recall on tests of memory. In another study with 19 female volunteers, 3 grams of glycine at bedtime was shown to reduce fatigue the next day.

How does glycine induce sleep in people with insomniac tendencies? Two proposed mechanisms of action have been suggested from studies on rats. The first is that glycine slightly decreases core body temperature in a manner similar to the natural decline that coincides with the onset of sleep; the second is that glycine increases the release of serotonin from the prefrontal cortex region of the brain. Serotonin is the feel-good neurotransmitter as well as the precursor to melatonin, the sleep hormone. In any case, taking glycine during the day does not cause drowsiness in humans, even in amounts up to 9 grams; no adverse effects have been observed with supplementation of 30 grams per day. My advice would be to start with 1 to 3 grams of glycine taken one hour before bedtime. The lower dose may work just as well if you consume collagen protein, rich in glycine, during the day.

If glycine alone is not quite doing the job for a patient, I will suggest adding in 1 gram of taurine and 300 mg magnesium. Often this combination leads to improved sleep within the first week, even in individuals who have been suffering from chronic insomnia.

Would collagen protein or gelatin work as well? According to Traditional Chinese Medicine, insomnia is an indication for the use of donkey-hide gelatin. Today, some holistic practitioners report that hydrolyzed collagen helps induce sleep, and they recommend combinations of collagen with other supplements like the amino acid tryptophan, a serotonin precursor, and the Indian spice turmeric, which reduces inflammation. As of now, there are no published studies on the effects of collagen protein or gelatin on sleep. If you do want try collagen protein for sleep, try gelatin, or look for a product that is enzymatically hydrolyzed without the use of acid (most good-quality products are), to avoid potentially consuming high levels of glutamates that can act as brain stimulants.

Detoxification

Detoxification and maintaining good antioxidant levels are key strategies in improving overall health. Glutathione, made up of glycine, cysteine, and glutamate, has one of the largest roles to play here—and collagen plays a big role in our body's production of glutathione. If you haven't heard of it before, get ready to learn about one of the hottest topics in the field of functional medicine.

When you think of antioxidants, do colorful fruits and vegetables first come to mind? Maybe you think of superfoods like pomegranates, goji berries, green tea, kale, garlic, rosemary, and turmeric, which you may include as a daily part of your diet. Great start. But did you know that one of the most powerful antioxidants of all is something your own body synthesizes?

That antioxidant is glutathione, so essential to life that it is found in virtually every cell in the body and is especially concentrated in our metabolic control center, the liver. Glutathione's job is to neutralize harmful molecules known as oxidants (reactive oxygen species) and other bad guys like free radicals, environmental toxins, and many drugs. In fact, the toxic effects of higher doses of certain medications, like acetaminophen, are due to the steep reductions in glutathione levels they cause. Glutathione also "reactivates" other antioxidants, including vitamins C and E, after they become oxidized.

After doing its cleanup work, glutathione gets "recycled," or restored to its active state from its oxidized state. But many things can and do interfere with the optimal recycling of glutathione, some under our control and some not. For example, simply getting older decreases our ability to recycle glutathione, and to make it in the first place. Unfortunately, irreversible damage can and does occur when our cells run short on glutathione. A shortage leads to higher levels of oxidative stress that causes our bodies to age more rapidly and become more susceptible to disease, in part by accelerating DNA damage. The good news is there is a lot that we can do to support optimal glutathione production.

Your diet plays a big part in how well you create, recycle, and utilize glutathione. Diets rich in fruits and vegetables, especially from the cabbage family and the berry family, are instrumental, as are optimal intakes of selenium, magnesium, folate, and other B vitamins. But while important, colorful fruits and vegetables are just a start. If you are guessing that collagen protein might be helpful, you would be right. To better understand how, you need to learn a little more about glutathione.

Glutathione is a tripeptide, or a short chain of three amino acids bonded together. The amino acids that make up glutathione are cysteine, glutamate, and glycine. When the body's demand for glutathione production increases, one of the best ways to meet that demand is by increasing the supply of the amino acids that glutathione is made from. For example, cases of liver toxicity caused by glutathione depletion (specifically caused by overdoses of acetaminophen)have been medically treated for decades with infusions of n-acetylcysteine (NAC), a more stable form of purified cysteine. NAC has also become a popular oral supplement for supporting liver health, albeit in much lower doses.

Maintaining Glutathione Levels with Collagen

So where does collagen protein fit into this picture? Collagen protein and gelatin are two of the best dietary sources of glycine. The synthesis of glutathione begins with cysteine and requires glycine (and magnesium and energy) to complete. Glycine and cysteine must be readily available for our bodies to make plenty of glutathione. Glutamate is rarely a problem, except during certain disease states or if overall protein intake is very low. Glycine is apt to be in limited supply after a meal rich in lean animal protein, especially without a balance of collagen-derived protein. There's an argument against some of those popular very high-protein diets!

After the age of 60, glutathione levels can drop to less than half of what our bodies produced in our thirties. Along with this, researchers have learned that glycine levels decline to the same extent and cysteine levels drop by one-quarter in older individuals. Researchers from Baylor College of Medicine suspected the age-related drop in glutathione levels could be restored. They gave eight volunteers between ages 60 and 75 the amino acids glycine and cysteine at doses equal to 0.1 gram per kilogram of body weight for two weeks. (This equates to 7.5 grams of each amino acid for the average 165-pound person, the amount of glycine contained in 28 grams or 5 rounded tablespoons of collagen protein.)

Remarkably, in just two weeks, the blood levels of glutathione in the elderly volunteers almost doubled, reaching those measured in younger individuals! There was also a significant decrease in markers of oxidative damage in the elderly, mirroring the lower levels in their juniors. The researchers concluded that marked decline in glutathione that occurs with aging can be corrected by supplementation with glycine and cysteine. Recall that there is an estimated shortfall of 8.5 to 10 grams of glycine per day in a majority of people's diets. So it is not at all surprising that providing 7.5 grams of glycine per day to elderly individuals would be very helpful.

Whatever your age, how can you apply these findings? Twenty-eight grams is a generous amount of collagen protein to consume each day, which I don't necessarily recommend to everyone, for reasons explained in Chapter 12. You may additionally want to consider supplementing with pure glycine. And while I cannot give specific dosage recommendations, 3 grams of glycine per day has already been proven efficacious for improving sleep and reducing anxiety.

In addition, you need to pay attention to the other half of the glutathione equation, the amino acid cysteine. One of the best food sources of cysteine is unheated whey protein, found in unpasteurized milk and now available in whey protein powders. Keep in mind when selecting a whey protein that it ideally should be low-temperature-processed and not an isolated whey protein, which is more widely available and often less expensive. It is best to mix up your whey beverage in a shaker bottle and avoid more than a quick spin in the blender, or the cysteine it contains may lose some of its biological activity.

Other Health-Supportive Roles

The list is a long one, so I will only touch on a few. Glycine is needed to make the heme part of our hemoglobin (the oxygen-transporting protein in our red blood cells), to make bile that helps break down fats in our diet, and to control the cellular gates that regulate the movement of electrolytes in our body. You will find more about supportive roles for glycine and weight loss in Chapter 8, blood sugar in Chapter 9, and pregnancy in Chapter 11.

The Role of Proline

In Chapter 3, you read that the body needs proline to synthesize new proteins and that this need surpasses that of all of the other amino acids. Proline is also the precursor to the amino acid arginine, which produces nitric oxide so the blood can flow more efficiently through our vessels. Arginine is important for male reproductive functioning, specifically in maintaining good sperm counts and motility. Good to know that collagen protein is 9 percent arginine as well!

Most protein-sufficient diets supply plenty of proline because it is found in all foods that contain protein; dairy and collagen protein are two of the best sources. Because it is so widespread in the diet, it is thought to be unlikely that a person is proline-deficient. Proline also works in all the same places that glycine does: helping form collagen, regenerating cartilage, forming connective tissue, repairing skin damage and wounds, healing the gut lining, and repairing joints.

In the early phases of wound healing, the levels of proline in a wound are at least 50 percent higher than those in the blood, which indicates that proline is actively transported into a healing wound. Proline and hydroxyproline work together to stabilize the collagen triple helix as new collagen is laid down in a wound. Rats fed proline-enriched diets showed no change in the rate of healing or the strength of a healed wound, whereas studies in humans and in rats both have shown that arginine supplementation enhances collagen deposition and improves the healing of wounds. Proline appears to have immune modulating, anti-inflammatory, and blood sugar–regulating effects. You will find more about this last property in Chapter 9.

CHAPTER 11

Collagen at Every Age, Every Stage

By now you appreciate how your skin, bones, joints, digestive tract, blood sugar, and heart can benefit from a diet rich in collagen protein. You're probably excited to see firsthand the benefits from your own daily collagen regimen. Like me, you'll become convinced that collagen protein is important for everyone who wants to fend off the signs of aging. However, it may come as a surprise that collagen protein is not just for adults!

In this chapter, I'll explain how a diet rich in collagen protein is beneficial even before we are born, continuing into childhood, and throughout our entire lives. Collagen protein is especially valuable during periods of growth and development and not just during periods of repair and recovery. I will begin with a few potential benefits of collagen protein for individuals in their senior years. Then I will focus the rest of the chapter on the importance of collagen protein through the other stages of life.

If You Are 55 Years or Older

You have already learned about the benefits of consuming collagen protein for more youthful skin, bones, and joints. And in Chapter 10, you learned that supplementation with the amino acids glycine and cysteine increased the levels of the body's all-important antioxidant glutathione in older individuals. Their glutathione levels doubled, rivaling the levels of their youthful counterparts in just two short weeks. This is exciting news, because there is a strong link between higher levels of oxidative stress and age-related illness, including cognitive decline, immune deficiencies, increased DNA damage, diabetes, and vision disorders. A combination of whey protein and collagen protein can be a great source of both of these difficult-to-obtain amino acids.

Collagen might just slow down the cognitive changes that go along with getting older. Although not yet studied in humans, marine collagen peptides facilitated learning and memory acquisition in older female mice. Chinese scientists discovered that when these mice were fed collagen peptides, they were able to perform equally as well as young mice on tests of spatial learning and memory. Although we are not the same as mice (but we do share almost 90 percent of their genetic code), female mice were selected because Alzheimer's disease is two to three times more common in women than in men after age 65. The scientists attributed the enhanced performance of the older mice to the improvements in antioxidant activity and the expression of brain-protective proteins seen with the collagen peptides. The amount of marine collagen peptides that gave the best results was 0.44 percent by weight of the mice's food. Assuming that the average woman consumes between 4 and 5 pounds of food per day and 20 percent of that is water (given a 2,000-calorie diet), we can estimate that 7 to 8 grams of marine collagen peptides would be an equivalent daily dose for humans.

Collagen Protein from the Very Start

While clearly beneficial in our senior years, collagen protein intake is equally if not even more important during another stage of life: fetal development. Even if you're well past your child-bearing years, please read on, as you may be able to share this helpful information with expectant parents.

Many women come to see me with hormonal problems, infertility, or pregnancy complicated by obesity or poor blood sugar control. The women I don't see anywhere nearly as often are those that do not experience problems conceiving or carrying a baby to term. This is a real shame, because all women can benefit from a thorough review of their diet by a knowledgeable dietitian or nutritionist before, during, and after pregnancy. Whether pregnant or trying to conceive, my patients consistently tell me how valuable the information I shared with them was and how glad they were to have met with me. In the words of one mother-to-be, "I didn't know what I didn't know."

Unfortunately, many women have gaps in their prenatal nutrition despite following the recommended dietary guidelines and receiving the best obstetrical care. Could these gaps lead to problems for a woman or her baby? Based on the growing body of research in reproductive nutrition, the potential is there. It is not uncommon for women before, during, and after pregnancy to underconsume or have low levels of several vitamins and minerals. Maternal undernutrition may be more prevalent in developed countries than the medical community recognizes. Insufficient intakes of vitamin A, vitamin D, vitamin B6, biotin, choline, zinc, iron, iodine, glycine, and/or omega-3 fats are not uncommon. While outright birth defects may not result, a shortage of one or more of these nutrients could adversely impact a child, potentially contributing to physical or mental health challenges at birth and over his or her lifetime. This is still a controversial theory, but as the research expands on the developmental origins of disease in the field of epigenetics (how the environment impacts our genes), I believe we will continue to see relationships between undernutrition and disease revealed.

My goal is to see all women be fully nourished during the critical life stages of pregnancy and lactation. In my practice, one of the most frequent recommendations I make to pregnant patients is that they consume more collagen protein. They are surprised to learn that daily servings of skin-on organic chicken, gelatin dishes, and soups made with bone broth are important parts of their prenatal diet. And I have yet to meet with an expectant mother who was already in the habit of eating these nourishing foods prior to our first appointment.

One of the main reasons collagen protein appears to be essential during pregnancy is, once again, that little amino acid glycine. According to nutritional scientists, "the shortage of glycine may become serious in conditions such as pregnancy." What might "serious" mean for a pregnant woman and her baby? Pregnancy creates a higher demand for glycine due to the increased collagen and elastin synthesis taking place in the expanding uterus and stretching skin. As a result, glycine may become a limiting factor for protein synthesis in the developing fetus: Without enough available glycine, there is the possibility that fetal growth will be restricted, albeit to an unknown extent. Additionally, in studies on pregnant rats, glycine supplementation reversed the high blood pressure and the blood vessel dysfunction that occurred when they were fed lower-protein diets. These findings point to an important (pivotal, per the authors) role for dietary glycine in the adaptations required during pregnancy to support healthy maternal circulation.

Recall from Chapter 3 that some scientists consider glycine to be one of the conditionally essential amino acids because the human body cannot synthesize enough glycine to meet more than its most basic survival needs. There are numerous health benefits to consuming sufficient quantities of glycine through diet, and 10 grams per day appears to be about optimal. And while 10 grams may be sufficient for almost every healthy adult, it is almost certain that a moderately higher amount (perhaps around 15 grams) would be beneficial during pregnancy, especially during the second and third trimesters when the most rapid growth occurs.

To better understand the role of glycine, we need to look at it in the context of the overall diet. It is generally recommended that a woman consume an additional 25 grams of protein per day during the second and third trimesters of pregnancy, or a total of 71 grams per day. Much more protein than this is not advisable. High-protein diets that exceed 20 percent of calories from protein can impair fetal growth, according to a 2013 review of the research.[9] And an excess of the amino acid methionine relative to glycine is not optimal either. Too much methionine not only increases the need for glycine, but may lead to other undesirable effects on the child's long-term physiology.

Where would an excess of methionine come from? From high-protein diets that are often thought of as healthy, and especially ones with predominantly lean muscle protein, like boneless, skinless chicken breast and lean boneless meat. So whether it is the total amount of protein or methionine, or the ratio of methionine to glycine consumed, it is important to make sure that the sources of protein are balanced, avoiding too little or too much. Nutritionists often refer to this as the "Goldilocks Principle," and it can be applied to almost any nutrient, supplement, or food that we consume.

---

9 For the typical 5-foot, 5-inch, 150-pound female, 20 percent of calories equates to 100 grams of protein when consuming 2,000 calories in the first trimester, and 120 grams of protein when consuming 2,400 calories in the third trimester.

Of course, collagen protein, although an excellent source of glycine and other amino acids, is just one component of a nourishing diet! When I am asked what the perfect meal for a pregnant woman is, I answer: a great homemade soup made with collagen-rich bone broth; 1 to 2 ounces of meat, poultry, organ meat, or safe seafood; 1 ounce of soft-cooked tendons, such as in the traditional Vietnamese dish pho; plenty of fresh leafy greens; a small potato or sweet potato; a half-cup of a favorite type of legume; a whole egg or, even better, two egg yolks; a bit of seaweed rich in iodine; and a handful of cilantro or other green herbs. On the side would be a fermented vegetable like sauerkraut. This would be accompanied by a good source of calcium such as a grass-fed cheese or yogurt, along with a fresh fruit for dessert, topped off by a little sunshine for vitamin D. Come to think of it, this is a perfect meal for just about anybody, at any time!

RECOVERY AFTER DELIVERY

Stretch marks happen when a women's belly expands faster than her skin can keep up with, causing the collagen and elastin fibers in the skin to break. Because collagen protein has been shown to increase the skin's elasticity, it just might minimize the appearance of those annoying stretch marks. Other than not gaining excessive weight during pregnancy, medical experts don't know how to prevent stretch marks. Collagen protein in the context of a nourishing diet could be your best defense.

Elastin: The "Other" Connective Protein

Elastin is the body's "elastic protein," and together with collagen, forms all of the body's connective tissue. Elastin is approximately 30 percent glycine and 15 percent proline. Like collagen, elastin consists of chains of amino acids networked by cross-links, but it lacks collagen's unique triple-helix structure. Elastin is one thousand times more flexible than collagen, although not nearly as strong. Because of its amazing ability to stretch and recoil, elastin is essential for the parts of the body that move and flex, allowing them to "bounce back" to their original shape. Less abundant in the body than collagen, elastin is concentrated in the lungs, skin, and ligaments, and the arteries coming off the heart. This makes sense when you consider the expansion and contraction that occurs as we take deep breaths, the suppleness and springiness of our skin, the plasticity that the ligaments connecting our bones exhibit as we move and stretch, and the resilience of blood vessels to handle the force of blood being pumped out of our hearts.

You can get an idea of the quality of the elastin in your skin by pinching yourself and watching how quickly your skin snaps back to its original shape. This won't happen where there is significant scarring due to the loss of elastin. After early childhood, human tissues synthesize few new elastin proteins, so scars are made predominantly of less-flexible collagen protein. Scientists are pursuing ways of delivering elastin protein directly to skin healing from burns to see if they eventually can reproduce normal skin flexibility.

In adults, existing elastin is replaced by newly synthesized elastin at a rate of just 1 to 2 percent each year, making elastin one of the longest-lasting proteins in our entire body. (The collagen in cartilage tissue turns over extremely slowly as well, with a half-life of almost 120 years, compared with the half-life of the collagen in the average adult's skin of about 15 years.) Because elastin is replaced so slowly, when significant damage occurs to tissues rich in elastin, such as a deep cut to the skin, there is often some degree of permanent injury.

During the developmental periods of life, elastin synthesis is anything but slow. In pregnancy, the simultaneous rapid growth of the developing fetus and the expansion of the woman's uterus requires that elastin be created faster than at any other stage of life. This accelerated production demands more of the substances that elastin is made from, predominantly glycine. In order to supply the fetus, the placenta both transports glycine from the mother's bloodstream and synthesizes glycine from another amino acid with assistance of the B vitamin folate. As stated previously, consuming collagen protein, in any of its forms, can be an ideal way to increase the amount of glycine in a mother's bloodstream.

Why Your Child Needs Collagen

You now have an idea of how incredibly long the elastin in your body hangs around. Another way of looking at this is to consider the half-life of elastin, or the amount of time it takes to turn over exactly one-half of all of the elastin in our bodies. That half-life is estimated to be a whopping 74 years! This means that in an average person's lifetime, half of their elastin will *never* be replaced. Clearly our body's elastin protein, first synthesized before we were born and continuing as we grow in size and stature, needs to withstand the physical stresses and strains of a lifetime. So it makes sense that the elastin laid down in early life should be the best quality possible.

Anecdotally, it seems to be more common today for children to exhibit signs of lax ligaments. During my walks on a popular recreation trail, I often observe adolescents and teenagers who appear to be training for a sport under the guidance of a coach or parent. It is not unusual to notice that their knees are out of alignment, their toes point inward, or they generally look somewhat floppy. A medical doctor has written her similar observations, calling them "classic signs of weak collagen." Like me, she believes the problem is not always due to low levels of physical activity, but to decreased collagen and elastin strength. This doctor's advice is the same as mine: To develop and maintain strong joints that are resistant to injury over the course of a lifetime, children must combine the stimulus of regular exercise with a collagen- and elastin-building diet.

Because elastin is intended to last for a lifetime, the body's production of new elastin dwindles after puberty. Due to the unique nature of its cross-link bonds, elastin can only be made when the body is replete with growth factors and hormones that direct its synthesis. This occurs during fetal development, childhood growth spurts, and adolescence.

When we eat animal proteins in the traditional ways, for example oxtail soup instead of a hamburger, headcheese instead of pork loin, or sardines with skin and bones instead of a fish filet, we ingest plentiful amounts of glycine and proline and other needed nutrients. This balance of amino acids supports the myriad of biological process, including the optimal growth and development of a child's body. If your child is involved in sports, providing them with foods rich in collagen protein or a collagen protein supplement could potentially prevent joint and connective tissue (ligaments and tendons) injuries now and joint deterioration in the future. Even if he or she prefers non-athletic activities, foods rich in collagen protein are a sound nutritional investment in his or her long-term health and mobility.

If you are well beyond your teenage years, you may be thinking the opportunity to protect or improve your ligament or joint health has passed you by. But while you cannot renew or replace the elastin in any part of your body by eating collagen, you can possibly prevent further deterioration. We know this is possible for the cartilage in joints, as we learned in Chapter 6.

Studies on the impact of collagen protein consumption over an individual's lifetime do not exist in the modern scientific literature. These studies would be virtually impossible to conduct due to the variation in individuals' diets over time and the prohibitive cost involved. What has been observed and documented by early nutrition pioneers are the sturdy builds of indigenous populations that never abandoned their nourishing traditional diets: diets rich in collagen protein and other body-building nutrients. These are too many nutrients to mention here, but in Chapter 14, I will cover the "other" foods and nutrients you need to round out your collagen-rich diet.

CHAPTER 12

How Much Collagen Protein Is Right for You?

Convinced by now that adding collagen protein to your diet is something you can benefit from? Great, but before you start mixing collagen protein or gelatin into everything you eat and drink, you'll want to keep a few things in mind.

First, collagen protein cannot replace the other sources of protein in your diet, because it lacks the essential amino acid tryptophan and contains only small amounts of the essential amino acid cysteine. So if you add collagen to your breakfast smoothie, make sure that you also use another protein source (whey, pea, egg, or rice protein, for example). If you like to make a one-bowl meal of soup, as I do, don't just serve a bowl of bone broth and vegetables; be sure to add some meat, chicken, or fish, cooked dried beans, cheese, tofu, or even a whole egg.

Second, you can actually have too much of a good thing, and that includes collagen protein. Let's look at the reasons why you don't want to go overboard with collagen protein or gelatin.

Other than the rare occurrence of an allergic reaction and the occasional complaint of heaviness in the stomach (which can be avoided by properly hydrating the supplements), there are no documented adverse side effects of consuming *normal* daily amounts of collagen protein. In 1975, gelatin, and by extension collagen protein, was approved to be "Generally Recognized as Safe" by the U.S. Food and Drug Administration. In animal studies, doses of hydrolyzed collagen equivalent to human intakes of about 100 grams per day did cause some kidney changes, but no other toxic effects have been observed. In one very small study with six people whose entire daily protein intake was in the form of collagen, half of the group experienced cardiac arrhythmias. Finally, in severe weight-loss diets supplying fewer than 500 calories per day in the form of only collagen protein, without any vitamins or minerals, a few deaths have occurred.

So, what is a *reasonable yet effective* amount of collagen to consume?

In general, to realize benefits, it is best to take 2.5 grams of high-quality collagen peptides daily, in addition to a maximum of 20 grams of collagen protein in the form of food and supplements, though I'd say between 10 to 15 grams per day is the sweet spot. When consuming more than 12 grams per day, it would be a good idea to split it between two meals. Collagen protein should not replace the other sources of protein in your diet to any great extent. My advice would be to review the chapter(s) on problems you want to address; you will find that almost all of the cited studies include the daily dosages tested. There are, however, a couple of caveats, discussed below.

Kidney Stones in Your Past?

If you are prone to kidney stones, you will want to increase the sources of collagen protein in your diet very gradually and very carefully. The reason is that both collagen and gelatin can generate oxalates in the body that get excreted in the urine, a prime trigger for the formation of a stone.

Nine out of ten kidney stones are made of calcium oxalate crystals, which form when the levels of oxalic acid in the urine become elevated. Most sufferers of recurrent kidney stones are instructed to limit or avoid foods high in oxalates, like spinach, beets, black tea, and worst of all, rhubarb. While this is usually very effective, only one-quarter to one-half of the oxalates excreted into the urine by the kidneys come from food or beverages.

The remainder comes from the breakdown of the amino acid hydroxyproline. Remember that hydroxyproline is one of the amino acids we find in great abundance in both collagen protein and gelatin; a major source of hydroxyproline in our bodies comes simply from the daily turnover of our body's own collagen. Much of this excess hydroxyproline is converted to glycine (and used for other beneficial purposes); the remainder is turned into oxalate and glycolate and is excreted by the kidneys via the urine. Since we naturally break down 2 to 5 grams of our own collagen each day, 1 to 3 mg of oxalates are generated from these conversions. This amount is not thought to present an increased risk for stone formation for a well-hydrated person who does not have a preexisting defect in oxalate metabolism.

But if you have ever suffered from kidney stones, you need to be aware of the results of a small study of male and female volunteers who consumed three different sources of proteins over a five-day period. They ate either a self-selected diet; a diet providing 10 grams of whey protein at each of three meals (30 grams total, representing 25 percent of the daily protein intake); or a diet providing 10 grams of gelatin at each of three meals (also 30 grams total, and 25 percent of the daily protein intake). When this last group consumed the gelatin protein, it caused the excretion of oxalates in the urine to increase 43 percent over the self-selected and whey protein diets. None of these volunteers had a history of kidney stones, and none experienced a kidney stone episode during this short study. However, an increase in urinary oxalates of this magnitude could be a cause for concern by those who are already at risk for kidney stone formation.

Finally, just because you have never had a kidney stone does not mean that you are not at risk for elevated oxalates in the urine that could lead to a stone. Approximately 1 in 10 people will develop a kidney stone at some point in their lives. If you want to determine if you might be at risk, discuss with your doctor getting your urine checked for the presence of calcium oxalate crystals, ideally very soon after you have consumed your usual amount of collagen protein or gelatin. Together, you can determine if you are at higher risk for kidney stones and if you may need to limit your intake of collagen protein to no more than around 10 grams per day, spread between meals.

Getting Headaches and Not Sleeping as Well as You Used To?

Collagen protein may not be a match for you if you have a sensitivity to one or more of its primary amino acids. One that seems to be particularly problematic is glutamic acid. Glutamic acid is essentially the same thing as glutamate, which is the most abundant neurotransmitter in our brains. Glutamate stimulates neurons in the brain and in this way sends messages, allowing us to think and learn and develop memory. It is generally bound up in the proteins we eat and hence slowly released with digestion. Alternatively, it can enter our bloodstream quickly if the protein we have consumed is hydrolyzed, such as collagen peptides or long-cooked broth. If we suddenly have too much free glutamate in our bodies, there is a chance that it can cross into our brain and overstimulate it. This is why, for some, consumption of collagen peptides, broth, and even gelatin[10] result in headaches and sleeplessness.

But something else is at play here beyond a high influx of glutamate from the food we eat. In general, if we have a well-functioning "blood brain barrier," the free glutamates we eat won't affect us negatively. The blood brain barrier consists of a layer of cells that controls what can and cannot cross into the brain. It seems that, like leaky gut, there is a condition that has been loosely referred to as "leaky brain." Both conditions are thought to result from chronic low-grade inflammation caused by a number of things: infections, toxins, and even the bad stuff that slips through a leaky gut!

Homemade broths can be high in glutamates, especially the longer they are cooked because more free amino acids are released. If you find you are experiencing changes in your sleeping patterns or are developing even low-grade headaches, stop all sources of collagen protein immediately, perhaps with the exception of the skin on fish and chicken and the cartilage on bones. If your symptoms resolve, this is a good indication that you may not tolerate free glutamates.

---

10   Great Lakes Gelatin company states that their products, gelatin, and hydrolyzed collagen are low in free glutamates.

It would be a leap to assume you have leaky brain, and since there is no medical test for it, a conventional doctor might not be of much help here. I suggest you see if removing foods that can contribute to leaky gut, such as grains containing gluten, stopping all alcohol and unnecessary medications, and adding a good probiotic allows you to tolerate small amounts of collagen peptides. If the problems resume, seek out a good functional or holistic practitioner. Several other foods are naturally high in glutamates, including Parmesan cheese, tomatoes, mushrooms, and anchovies. Anything that heightens the taste of a food (outside of salt, pepper, herbs, and spices) is a possibility, so be aware if you think you are experiencing a reaction to collagen protein.

Broths can also be high in histamine, to which some people experience symptoms of histamine intolerance, including headaches and insomnia, anxiety, flushing, and other symptoms similar to seasonal allergies. This intolerance is thought to be due to a higher responsiveness of the body's histamine receptors and/or a defect in the body's ability to break down histamine. Histamine is also released during allergic reactions, and it serves normal physiological functions in the gut and in the brain. Like glutamate, it acts as a neurotransmitter. The same advice for suspected glutamate intolerances applies here, but I would just add to make sure your meat, fish, and chicken is very fresh, whether cooked into broth or prepared in any other way.

CHAPTER 13

Collagen Supplements: Frequently Asked Questions

Ready to include more collagen protein in your diet but find it difficult to eat foods naturally rich in collagen protein on a daily basis? Bone broth, poultry, and fish skin (not to mention fried pork rinds!), the connective tissue attached to meaty bones, and the soft bones in canned fish are certainly a great way to go, but sometimes they can be hard to fit into a dietary routine. Because collagen protein should be consumed on a daily basis to achieve consistent results, supplements are the ideal choice for many people.

In the previous chapters you learned about the many different types of collagen protein—bovine, marine, porcine, or poultry; hydrolyzed/peptides or gelatin—and may have selected one that you think best matches your unique health goals. When purchasing a collagen supplement, you now need all the details on what the safest and most effective choice for you is. In this chapter, I'll provide answers to the questions most frequently asked about collagen protein supplements.

1. What are the differences between collagen hydrolysate, collagen peptides, and gelatin? What about bone broth?

2. How do I select the best types of collagen and gelatin protein?

3. Is it important that my collagen protein be non-GMO, organic, and/or pastured-raised?

4. Are there vegetarian, kosher, or halal collagen proteins?

5. What is the minimum amount of collagen protein I need to take daily to see results?

6. Are there any downsides or contraindications to collagen protein consumption? Is it possible to consume too much collagen or gelatin?

7. Can I take tablets or capsules, or do I need to mix a powder into something I eat or drink?

8. Can I take collagen protein with food or should it be on an empty stomach?

9. What other ingredients in collagen protein should I be looking for?

10. Can I mix collagen protein into any liquid, hot or cold?

11. Can I cook or bake with collagen protein?

12. How should I store collagen protein, and how long does it keep?

13. Why do I hear from the media and other sources that collagen protein is not what it claims to be?

1. What are the differences between collagen hydrolysate, collagen peptides, and gelatin? What about bone broth?

As discussed in Chapter 3, all collagen protein products are derived from the same raw material: intact collagen proteins. "Collagen protein" is a catch-all term that is used for the class of proteins derived mainly from the hide, skin, bone, cartilage, tendon, and hooves of a land animal, or the skin, scales, and fins of a sea-dwelling animal. Gelatin is what I'll call the "first pass" processing of collagen protein, heated long enough to relax its twisted conformation but not so long as to degrade its lengthy amino acid structure. This is basically the same thing that happens when you make a slow-cooked bone broth that yields a gelled product upon cooling. If your broth doesn't congeal, it may mean it is low in collagen protein, or it may be that you just cooked it too fast or too long. Overcooking can easily occur when making a fish-based broth. Because fish gelatin is less cross-linked, it has lower thermal stability compared to poultry gelatin, which in turn has lower thermal stability compared to cow and pig gelatins.

"Collagen peptides" and "collagen hydrolysates" are terms used to describe gelatin that has been further processed. The gelatin has been digested using an enzymatic or chemical process to yield very small fragments of collagen protein. These fragments are so small that they are unable to form a hydrophilic (water-attracting) gel when dissolved in a hot liquid and then cooled. Although they cannot form a gel, they will readily dissolve into any temperature beverage or into any food with a high water content. Once absorbed by our digestive tract, collagen peptides/hydrolysates turn into biologically active molecules with special benefits. Note that the generic term "collagen protein" can be used to describe both the hydrolysate and peptide forms, but most products are now simply labeled as "collagen peptides."

Because gelatin is hydrophilic, it forms what are called "colloids" in the digestive tract. This seems to be one of the reasons behind the gut-healing and digestion-supporting properties of homemade broths and soups. We covered this in depth in Chapter 6. Bone broth has been around for millennia, yet just in the past decade has its status been elevated to one of the trendiest superfoods out there. I've included surprisingly simple recipes for you on page 169. If you decide instead to buy it, you will find a few caveats and tips on how to improve a store-bought broth (page 74). Real bone broth has more active ingredients in it than does collagen protein (including glycosaminoglycans and minerals), but there are no published trials on its benefits. Bone broths can vary widely in the amount of the key amino acids that support collagen synthesis and may or may not yield the results seen in studies using collagen peptides.[11] There was one study that seemed to indicate that bone broth is high in lead, but the amount was well under the EPA limits for lead in drinking water, so unlikely to pose harm. Further, glycine has been shown to mitigate the effects on lead in rat studies. Use bones from pastured animals raised in rural areas whenever possible.

2. How do I select the best types of collagen and gelatin protein?

You will probably want to review the chapter(s) in this book that focus on your most immediate health goals—perhaps better skin and nails, more comfortable digestion, less joint pain, etc. Once you have identified the type(s) of collagen protein indicated in the studies in those chapters, you will want to consider the source. Brands that I trust for my patients include Vital Proteins, Ancient Nutrition, and Sports Nutrition Research, as well as Life Extension and Designs

---

11 R. D. Alcock, G. C. Shaw, and L. M. Burke, "Bone broth unlikely to provide reliable concentrations of collagen precursors compared to supplemental sources of collagen used in collagen research." *International Journal of Sport Nutrition and Exercise Metabolism.* https://journals.humankinetics.com/doi/abs/10.1123/ijsnem.2018-0139?url_ver=Z39.88-2003&rfr_id=ori:rid:crossref.org&rfr_dat=cr_pub%3dpubmed.

for Health (both combination products), as they generally meet the criteria described below.

Traditionally, collagen and gelatin have been derived from land animals like pigs and cows; the term "porcine" means sourced from a pig, "bovine" from a cow. A third increasingly popular type of collagen, "marine collagen" is sourced from wild-ocean or farm-raised fish. The first decision you need to make is whether to choose porcine, bovine, or marine collagen. (Chicken collagen is available for targeted purposes, see page 67.) Obviously, the choice is immediately narrowed if you do not eat one or more of these foods. If you should have concerns relating to allergic reactions, religious beliefs, ethical choices, or just knowing where food you eat comes from, it's a good idea to contact the manufacturer to be completely safe.

So which is best: porcine, bovine, or marine collagen? I've personally used all three types of collagen peptides, and I have used porcine gelatin, as it is the most widely available—Great Lakes and Knox Gelatin both are porcine products. A couple of studies I read mentioned, without further evaluation, that there is a potential risk for mad cow disease with bovine collagen. I think this is probably an extremely low risk if you follow the other guidelines on selecting collagen products given here.

3. Is it important that my collagen protein be non-GMO, organic, and/or pastured-raised?

If you are already on or want to start a collagen or gelatin regimen, you'll want to consider this. Many collagen products are obtained from animals raised in what are called concentrated animal feeding operations or CAFOs, a term coined by the USDA. If you don't know the issues surrounding CAFOs, I urge you to do a little research on the topic. Not all of these operations are inhumane to the livestock, but most of the practices would surprise and even disappoint many a meat-eater. I have tried to purchase free-range organic meat and poultry as often as possible for the past 20 or so years, but until recently, it had not occurred to me that my collagen choices should meet those same standards.

Looking at the clean white powder that is collagen protein, the connection to an animal is not readily made, unlike a steak or a chicken leg. You have heard "you are what you eat," but have you heard "you are what you eat eats?" I can't take credit for this new adage, but it resonates with me. If you eat CAFO-raised animals given feed containing pesticides and other potentially harmful additives, you effectively get a higher concentration of these unwanted chemicals because of the effect of bioaccumulation.

One particularly problematic pesticide added to animal feed is glyphosate. Remember the little amino acid that can, glycine? Recall that it makes up about one-third of collagen protein. Well, it appears that the glyphosate molecule, which looks chemically a lot like glycine, is able to sneak in and replace glycine during the synthesis of collagen and other proteins. While for many proteins this hardly matters, glycine is uniquely required for some proteins in our bodies to function properly. Myosin, a protein in our muscles that is responsible for movement, appears to be one that could be affected by a substitution of glyphosate for glycine; our own collagen could well be another.

The idea that our own collagen (and the collagen protein we consume!) might contain high levels of glyphosate has been brought to the forefront by Dr. Stephanie Senff. Dr. Senff is a research scientist at the MIT Computer Science and Artificial Intelligence Laboratory, and has published more than two dozen papers on the relationship between nutritional deficiencies, dietary toxins, and health. She is working to unravel the reasons we are seeing rapid rises in many chronic conditions, especially allergies, rheumatoid arthritis, osteoporosis, and autoimmune diseases, as well as less common ones like autism. According to Senff, evidence points to glyphosate substituting for glycine as a big contributor.

Bottom line: Eat organic and grass-fed foods as much as possible, including your supplements, especially those that come from animals, and especially collagen protein. At a minimum, look for the term "non-GMO" on the label. This means that the animal was *not* fed GMO corn and soybeans, which typically contain a lot of pesticide residues, especially glyphosate. Never assume a product is non-GMO.

Note that Verisol collagen peptides do not appear to be pasture-raised, but it is a non-GMO product according to one supplier, Designs for Health.

4. Are there any vegetarian, kosher, or halal collagen products?

Collagen protein and gelatin come solely from animals—land and sea—and therefore do not meet the requirements of a vegan, lacto, or lacto-ovo vegetarian diet. Neither eggs nor dairy contain collagen protein, nor does any plant food. Having read about all of collagen's benefits, however, you may want to consider making an exception to consume collagen protein, especially if you follow a vegetarian diet for health reasons. If this is the case, I would encourage you to give marine collagen a try.

Kosher-certified collagen peptides are available from Innate Vitality and Vital Proteins, and other companies may offer some as well. BioCell manufactures a halal-certified chicken collagen; another halal product is sold under the label Bee-natural and is organic and derived from fish.

5. What is the minimum amount of collagen peptides I need to take daily to see results?

This varies between individuals according to sex, weight, degree of muscle and bone mass, and desired outcome. The lowest effective dose in the studies reviewed was 2.5 grams, but that tested a targeted collagen peptide, Verisol, on skin outcomes. I would use the amount the manufacturer recommends for at least one to two months before adjusting on my own. You may wish to also eat foods naturally rich in collagen or gelatin protein to supplement your intake.

6. Are there any downsides or contraindications to collagen protein consumption? Is it possible to consume too much collagen or gelatin?

There are almost no downsides to collagen protein consumption unless you have an allergy to it; you fail to mix it up well in a fluid before consumption, which can result in stomach discomfort; you have kidney stones; and/or you consistently take more than the recommended dose on the product label. See Chapter 12 for more detail on dosing.

7. Can I take tablets or capsules or do I need to mix a collagen peptide powder into something I eat or drink?

Most of the available products come in a powder form because of the quantity needed to see results, usually 6 to 10 grams or more daily. Verisol collagen peptides are available in tablet form because the effective dose is relatively small at 2.5 grams daily.

8. Can I take collagen peptides with food or should I consume them on an empty stomach?

As always, refer to the label, but there is some evidence that consuming collagen peptides with a form of fermented dairy like yogurt or kefir could enhance their absorption.

9. What other ingredients in collagen protein should I look for?

Again, this depends on what your goals are. Some possibilities could be a flavor to create a beverage you enjoy or active ingredients like vitamins and minerals, hyaluronic acid, biotin, silica, aloe vera, or antioxidants such as polyphenols, green tea, and taurine. I would avoid collagen protein with vitamins and minerals if you are already taking other supplements that contain those ingredients, unless working closely with a nutritionist or other practitioner.

10. Can I mix collagen protein into any liquid, hot or cold?

If you want to mix collagen protein (in the form of collagen peptides) into a beverage of your choice, temperature of the liquid generally does not make a difference. Two things to consider: The powder may dissolve more quickly in something warm or hot, and other active ingredients may be temperature-sensitive. Always follow the product's label directions.

11. Can I cook or bake with collagen protein?

Yes, as long as the label indicates you can heat the product. Products containing vitamins are best not exposed to heat beyond room temperature. Gelatin is great for adding moisture to ground meats before cooking, and thickening sauces and gravies. Always pre-hydrate dry gelatin in a smaller amount of cool liquid to prevent clumping, then stir it into boiling liquid. Gelatin requires a minimum of 140°F to fully dissolve.

12. How should I store collagen protein, and how long does it keep?

Products have expiration dates on them, so you will want to refer to those. I have used collagen beyond the manufacturer's use-by date and have not had a problem, but I would advise you to only purchase what you can use by the expiration date. A container generally lasts about one month when taking it daily. Always store gelatin in a dry pantry or cabinet where the humidity is low, not in the refrigerator as it can absorb moisture and degrade, especially after it is opened. When purchasing collagen protein in pouches, you may want to transfer it to airtight containers.

13. Why do I hear in the media and from other sources that collagen protein is not what it is claimed to be?

There is always a high level of skepticism when a dietary supplement is promoted as having such a wide range of beneficial applications for beauty and wellness. But because the human diet used to contain much higher amounts of collagen protein than it does now, this is reason alone to consider including it in your own diet. While no reputable manufacturer can guarantee the results you are hoping for, a high-quality product should not cause adverse side effects unless you ignore any precautions on the label and those listed in this chapter. The biggest risk you might be taking is spending money (less than $100 in most cases) and not seeing the results you hoped for after a few months. Keep in mind that to see results, you must be prepared to take a product daily in the amount the manufacturer recommends, and you must continue to take the product for at least one to six months, depending on the desired outcome.

CHAPTER 14

Collagen's Supporting Cast

No nutrient acts in isolation, and dietary collagen protein is no exception.

While our bodies require the full array of essential nutrients, a few vitamins and minerals play starring roles in the formation and maintenance of our collagen. The ones we need to pay special attention to are the vitamins A, C, and biotin, and the minerals iron, zinc, copper, and perhaps silicon. You probably already know about the calcium and vitamin D combo for your bones, so we won't cover that here. There are also a myriad of nutraceuticals and herbs that are promoted for healthy collagen production in the body and some can be quite effective. Let's examine what both basic nutritional science and new research says about the strongest contenders for collagen-supporting vitamins and minerals.

Vitamin D

Vitamin D has been the darling of the nutrition world for more than a decade. Adequate levels are very important for strong bones because vitamin D is necessary for optimal calcium absorption. However, the science on its other roles in human health remains unsettled. Because vitamin D is a team player, paying attention to its mates, vitamins A and K2, is almost certainly part of the puzzle as to why vitamin D doesn't always hit a home run in studies on cancer and heart disease. To determine how much vitamin D is beneficial for you, I recommend reading *Vitamin K2 and the Calcium Paradox* by Kate Rheaume-Bleue and "Vitamin D Supplementation—Panacea or Potential Problem?" by yours truly.

Vitamin A and Zinc

Vitamin A and zinc are required by the cells that synthesize procollagen, the precursor to collagen. It is within these cells (fibroblasts in the skin or chondrocytes in the cartilage, for example) that the individual amino acid strands are first strung together, assembled by threes, and coiled into the procollagen triple helix. The procollagen is then exported out of the cells into the extracellular matrix, where the finishing touches that turn it into a mature collagen molecule are completed. It is in the extracellular matrix where each collagen molecule plays its part until it is selected for recycling, and the process of creating a new collagen molecule starts all over again.

Vitamin A communicates messages that regulate the cells synthesizing the procollagen. It also directs the cells that make up the epidermis. Without enough vitamin A in the diet, the ability to heal even superficial wounds is compromised, the skin becomes "keratinized" with small hard bumps forming on the surface, and even the glands that produce sweat and moisturizing oils shrink.

Zinc is required to make the protein that carries vitamin A from the liver to the other parts of the body where it is needed. The enzymes that perform the normal degrading and remodeling of collagen also depend on zinc, which becomes especially important during wound healing. Without enough zinc, the cross-links between the collagen molecules are impaired, weakening the skin's strength. Zinc also stimulates bone collagen synthesis, and in zinc deficiency, the normal time for bone collagen to turn over can triple. And speaking of bones, vitamin A acts in concert with vitamin D to balance the equally important processes of bone synthesis and bone breakdown.

Iron and Vitamin C

Iron is required for the reaction that affixes hydroxyl groups to the amino acids proline and lysine in the procollagen. The hydroxyl groups then create the links that form as three strands of amino acids come together. It's vitamin C's job to "activate" both the iron molecules and the enzyme that facilitates the addition of the hydroxyl groups. The bone, skin, nails, and hair all require iron, even though the skin's requirement is fairly low. Increased breakdown of bone can occur even with a mild iron deficiency. Dry skin and lips, brittle nails, and hair loss are symptoms of low iron levels, especially in women. This is not surprising when you understand the role that iron plays in collagen formation.

Copper

Copper is required to create the normal cross-linking that further stabilizes mature collagen. It's fairly uncommon to have a copper deficiency as compared to a zinc deficiency; what is more typical is that these two minerals are out of balance. Copper deficiency can cause a malabsorption of iron, so the clinical picture begins to get quite complex. To avoid copper deficiency, do not supplement with zinc without adding copper; aim for 1 mg of copper for every 15 mg of zinc, and don't exceed 30 to 45 mg of zinc per day unless recommended by a knowledgeable practitioner.

Biotin

Most products formulated to improve the hair, skin, and nails contain very high doses of biotin; some contain collagen protein, zinc, and vitamin C. Do they work? Yes, according to reports I hear from my patients who have been consistently taking them. Is it the biotin? Could be, but published case reports indicate that there is little benefit to taking biotin when the adequate intake of 30 micrograms per day is met.

I tend to side with my patients here. However, it's entirely possible that some women with hair loss actually have biotin deficiencies because they don't eat one of the best sources of biotin: egg yolks. And cooked as well as raw egg whites contain a protein called avidin that can oppose the action of biotin in the body. (You may already know not to eat too many uncooked egg whites.)

Two warnings about high-dose biotin supplementation. One, it can interfere with some common blood tests, giving false results, so you should let your doctor know that you are taking it, or at least stop for a couple of weeks in advance. Two, some women have noted that it can make all of the hair on their body grow faster and thicker, not just the hair on their heads!

Silicon

Silicon supplements are promoted to improve skin, nails, and hair. The predominant mineral in nails is silicon. A combination of choline and silicon, called choline-stabilized orthosilicic acid, is touted as clinically proven. There have been a couple of human trials with this form of silicon, with improvements seen in skin and nails, and perhaps bone collagen. There is a question about whether safety with long-term use has been adequately demonstrated, and although silicon is found in food, its status as an essential trace mineral has not been established. On the other hand, lots of people report that they definitely see the improvements promised from taking stabilized orthosilicic acid.

Hyaluronic Acid

Right up there with collagen, oral and topical hyaluronic acid is marketed as the answer to moist, more youthful skin and better lubricated joints. Called the body's natural hydrator, this humectant, when used topically, draws moisture from the air into your skin and has an ability to hold up to 1,000 times its weight in water. Oral supplementation with hyaluronic acid has shown promising results in clinical trials for osteoarthritis, dry eyes, wound healing, and aging skin. Unfortunately, hyaluronic acid levels decline with age. I think when applied topically it is hard to go wrong with hyaluronic acid, but taken internally I would advise some caution. It appears that some of the available products contain "low-molecular weight" hyaluronic acid, when the body's own healthy form is actually a "high-molecular weight." Low-molecular weight could possibly trigger inflammation rather than reduce it and could even enhance the migration of tumors. This information is not widely known; I first became aware of it from a product information sheet published by Klaire Labs, a nutritional supplement company that manufactures quality products recommended by health professionals.

Antioxidants

Skin-targeting antioxidants, specifically grape-skin extract, coenzyme Q10, luteolin, and selenium, have been added to marine collagen peptides (combined in a single product called Celergen, not yet available in United States). This formulation was shown to increase dermal thickness and density, and enhance skin elasticity and sebum (oil) production after two months of daily administration. The formula was specifically designed to reduce the potential for a higher rate of oxidative stress that is known to occur with an induction of collagen synthesis. The researchers did note a significant reduction of a marker for elevated oxidation in the 41 volunteers at the completion of the study. Skin-surface oil, or sebum, is essential for skin smoothness, elasticity, moisture, and barrier protection. Because the body's production of sebum gradually declines starting around age 50, as well as in UV-induced premature skin aging, an increase was considered a beneficial outcome.

Astaxanthin

Astaxanthin is another potent antioxidant that can enhance the effects of collagen protein. More powerful than other types of carotenoids, astaxanthin is the plant pigment that gives salmon, shrimp, and lobster their characteristic reddish-orange color. Algae and krill (very tiny crustaceans) are two sources for astaxanthin in supplements. When 44 volunteers took 2 mg of astaxanthin along with 3 grams of collagen hydrolysate daily for 12 weeks, they had improved elasticity and a reduction of water loss in their photo-aged skin. At the same time, this combination supplement decreased the expression of genes that code for metalloproteinases, which is associated with slowing the breakdown of existing collagen.

I have not seen any studies that compared the effects of collagen peptides with and without krill, so it is too early to say if astaxanthin makes a significant difference in skin appearance. But it does seem to enhance physical endurance, encourage the body to burn more fat during exercise, and slow down the muscle loss that accompanies aging. For those reasons alone, it is worth a try as an additional supplement to your daily collagen protein.

Plants and Herbs

A number of plants have been shown to help with skin quality and recovery from environmental damage. Aloe vera is one of the most popular and has a long history of use in folk remedies. Aloe can either be taken internally or applied directly to the skin, and both methods have been shown to significantly increase the collagen content of healing wounds. Topical application almost doubled the rate of collagen synthesis, and oral supplementation increased it by two-thirds in animal studies. Japanese women who consumed 40 micrograms of purified aloe vera mixed into their yogurt every day for 12 weeks experienced significant improvements in skin hydration and elasticity. These visible improvements were associated with an increase in the synthesis of collagen and hyaluronic acid in their skin.

Gotu kola, known botanically as *Centella asiatica*, has a long history of use in Asia, where it grows wild in wetland areas. One of the ways it improves the health and recovery of skin is through the induction of type I collagen synthesis; it also stimulates hyaluronic acid production and increases growth factors during wound healing. Very dilute solutions (0.1 to 0.2 percent) of gotu kola are effective when applied to the skin; orally, daily doses between 1 and 24 mg per kilogram of body weight (equivalent to 75 to 1,800 mg of dry herb for a 165-pound person) are considered effective, but it is probably most effective when taken in extract form. Either applied to the skin or taken orally, gotu kola reduces the appearance of photo-aging, cellulite, and stretch marks, and facilitates the healing of scratches, burns, and wounds.

Calendula officinalis, an herbal preparation made from a variety of marigold native to the Mediterranean, has been traditionally used on the skin for its anti-inflammatory and wound-healing properties. Applying a gel or cream made from 7 percent calendula can significantly increase collagen synthesis; lower levels are ineffective and higher levels may exert skin-damaging effects.

While this list is far from exhaustive, I have covered some of the heavy-hitters among the available supplements to arrest or reverse damage to collagen, whether from aging, UV exposure, or years of perhaps not following the best diet. Start with a good collagen protein regimen, and then consider the appropriate add-ons.

PART 2

RECIPES

CHAPTER 15

Collagen: Easy and Delicious Ways to Get More

Getting more collagen protein in your diet doesn't have to be complicated. You may already be enjoying foods that are rich in collagen protein, and eating just one or two servings daily could go a long way toward meeting your needs. However, while high in collagen protein, these foods may not offer the same benefits of collagen peptides or bone broth.

Some of the more popular foods rich in collagen protein are:

- Beef tendon, in soups like pho

- Chicken wings (feet are even better!)

- Gelatin molds, savory, or made with fruit or herbal tea

- Oxtail

- Pigs or calf's food jelly

- Pork skins or pork rinds, preferably baked

- Poultry skin

- Salmon skin

- Soups made with bone broth

- Veal shank

Whether or not you eat any of these foods on a regular basis, you may still want to take collagen peptides daily. The easiest way to do this is to mix an unflavored collagen peptide powder into your coffee, tea, flavored water, or juice. You will probably find that stirring in one rounded tablespoon (about 6 grams) of collagen peptides is barely detectable.

My personal collagen regimen starts with a cup or two of bone broth and one or two small servings of a homemade gelatin "gummy" each day. I try to include one or the other at every meal because I find that the gut-restoring qualities of the broth and gelatin really do help my digestion. I also have noticed that I am rarely hungry between meals with this plan. My choice of collagen peptides is a supplement containing Verisol collagen peptides and Cynatine solubilized keratin (Hair, Skin & Nails Rejuvenation Formula with Verisol by Life Extension) because my focus is on protecting my skin and strengthening my nails. So far so good—my skin looks great, I have no joint pain, and my nails are becoming more flexible and seem to be growing faster. I am even sleeping better.

Besides mixing collagen peptides into your morning beverage, another easy option is to turn your daily protein shake into a collagen-packed superstar. And because collagen protein readily mixes into liquids, hot or cold, you can add it to any of these foods: soups, sauces, stews, chili, salad dressings, hot cereals, yogurt, kefir, dips, spreads, and even batters prior to baking. You will come up with your own favorite ways as you experiment with the recipes I've provided. Your family may benefit as well, and might not even realize that you are fortifying their favorite foods with the nutrition of collagen protein! According to one mother: "I sneak it into the family soup, casserole dishes, noodles, etc. They don't have a clue. My family needs connective tissue support, too!"

Speaking of "sneaking" collagen protein into favorite foods, here are a few ideas:

- Any soup or stew

- Mashed potatoes, sweet potatoes, or cauliflower

- Pancake or muffin batter

- Tomato sauce or other pasta sauces

- Scrambled eggs

- Tuna or chicken salad made with mayonnaise

- Dips, dressings, or spreads

- Milk, dairy or dairy-free, for cereal

- Yogurt or kefir

Start by stirring in 1 to 2 teaspoons per serving (½ to 1 cup) to see how you like the result and increase up to 1 tablespoon per cup.

A note on bone broths: None of the recipes in this book use bone broth powders—I have tried a few and have not liked the flavor. Always use homemade when you have it, or purchase a shelf-stable broth like Swanson's Organic or Kettle and Fire. There are also ready-made frozen bone broths, which are costlier than the shelf-stable ones but may be closer to homemade in nutrition and flavor.

For additional recipes, visit www.thecollagendietplan.com.

Omelet with Sweet Potato Twirls

You can add collagen peptides to any egg scramble; just make sure to dissolve the peptides in a small amount of liquid before adding to the eggs. These sweet potato twirls offer an alternative to the classic accompaniment of toast for those who follow a gluten-restricted diet.

Yield: 1 serving | Total Time: 15 to 20 minutes

1 tablespoon olive oil

1 medium sweet potato, peeled and spiralized or cut into thin strands

½ teaspoon salt, divided

1 rounded tablespoon collagen peptides

2½ tablespoons water

3 large eggs

pinch of black pepper

1 tablespoon butter

2 teaspoons chopped chives (optional)

1. Heat the olive oil in a large skillet over medium-high heat.

2. Add the sweet potato noodles and ¼ teaspoon of the salt, stirring to coat. Reduce the heat to medium for 6 to 7 minutes, lightly covering in between stirring the noodles once or twice each minute.

3. Transfer the sweet potato noodles to large bowl. Set aside.

4. In a small bowl, whisk the collagen peptides into the water, then whisk this into the eggs in a medium bowl, with ¼ teaspoon of the salt plus a pinch of pepper, beating the eggs until smooth and you see a few air bubbles.

5. In the same skillet, melt the butter over medium heat.

6. Pour in the egg mixture and swirl the pan. Leave for 20 seconds until the eggs begin to bubble.

7. Using a fork, draw in the sides of the eggs to the center while shaking the pan to redistribute the liquid to the edges. The omelet is done when still slightly soft in the middle.

8. Add the sweet potato noodles to one half of the omelet, then fold the other half over the top.

9. Slide onto a plate and top with chives if desired.

NUTRITION INFORMATION PER SERVING
Total Protein: 25g   Collagen Protein: 6g
Calories: 486   Carbohydrates: 25g   Fat: 5g   Fiber: 4g

Berry Oatmeal Bake

This is a simple recipe that quite possibly could become one of your family's favorite breakfast or snack foods. Substitute other seasonal fruits like sliced peaches or plums if desired. You can use a pumpkin spice blend for the combination of spices if desired.

Yield: 4 (1-cup) servings | Total Time: 40 minutes

butter or coconut oil for the pan	¼ cup collagen peptides
2 cups rolled oats	1 tablespoon coconut oil
1 teaspoon ground cinnamon	1 egg
½ teaspoon ground ginger	2 tablespoons honey
¼ teaspoon ground nutmeg	1½ cups almond milk
¼ teaspoon ground cloves	1 cup berries of choice

1. Preheat the oven to 350°F. Grease an 8 x 8-inch square baking pan with butter or coconut oil.

2. In a medium bowl, stir together the oats, cinnamon, ginger, nutmeg, cloves, and collagen peptides.

3. In a separate medium bowl, whisk together the coconut oil, egg, honey, and almond milk.

4. Combine the wet and dry ingredients. Fold in the berries with a spatula to prevent them from bursting.

5. Pour into the prepared pan and bake for 35 to 40 minutes, until the top is golden brown and the almond milk is completely absorbed.

6. Store in an airtight container in refrigerator.

NUTRITION INFORMATION PER CUP
Total Protein: 14g   Collagen Protein: 7g
Calories: 290   Carbohydrates: 42g   Fat: 8g   Fiber: 5

Pumpkin Protein Pancakes

High in protein and relatively low in carbohydrates, these are easy to make and are somewhat moister than regular pancakes, so you won't need much butter and syrup to enjoy them. I love that the taste reminds me of pumpkin pie. But if pumpkin pie isn't your favorite, you can substitute ½ cup apple-sauce for the canned pumpkin and cinnamon for the pumpkin pie spice. This is also a great way to use up leftover baked sweet potatoes; just be sure to mash them well first. I keep my pancakes small, about 4 inches in diameter, so I can stack three together for a delicious breakfast. One or two pancakes also make a nice dessert topped with a dollop of whole milk vanilla yogurt or a bit of whipped cream. They keep great in the fridge a for few days or in the freezer for a few months, so you may want to make a double batch! To make these pancakes gluten-free, simply use a gluten-free pancake mix. I like the King Arthur brand.

Yield: 8 pancakes | Total Time: 30 minutes

½ cup pancake mix

½ teaspoon pumpkin pie spice (or cinnamon and/or nutmeg)

½ teaspoon salt

½ teaspoon baking powder

4 whole eggs

1 cup ricotta cheese or whole milk

⅔ cup canned pumpkin

¼ cup hydrolyzed collagen or collagen peptides

1 tablespoon melted butter, ghee, or other oil for the pan

butter and real maple syrup, for serving

1. In a small bowl, stir together the pancake mix, pumpkin pie spice, salt, and baking powder.

2. In a medium bowl, beat the eggs and whisk in the ricotta cheese or milk, canned pumpkin, and collagen powder. Mix in the dry ingredients just until combined, leaving no obvious lumps.

3. Warm a skillet or electric griddle over medium-high heat and lightly grease with butter, ghee, or oil.

4. Ladle pancake batter onto the cooking surface. These pancakes are very moist and will need a slightly longer time to cook thoroughly as compared to a standard pancake, so don't turn too soon. You will know when they are ready to flip when the batter in the center begins to set up, 4 to 5 minutes per side..

5. Serve with butter and syrup as desired. Leftovers (if you have any!) are great reheated in a microwave.

NUTRITION INFORMATION PER PANCAKE
Total Protein: 22g   Collagen Protein: 8g
Calories: 270   Carbohydrates: 15g   Fat: 15g   Fiber: 1g

Honey-Banana Protein Pancakes

If you don't have coconut flour, it can be replaced in this recipe with coconut flakes processed until fine in a food processor or blender. Serve these pancakes with butter, honey, and bananas, as desired.

Yield: 6 large pancakes | Total Time: 45 minutes

3 large eggs

½ cup full-fat yogurt

1 cup mashed ripe bananas

2 tablespoons raw honey (optional)

2 tablespoons fresh lemon juice

1 tablespoon coconut oil, plus more for cooking

1 teaspoon vanilla extract

¼ cup plus 2 tablespoons coconut flour

¼ cup collagen peptides

1 teaspoon baking powder

¼ teaspoon baking soda

1 teaspoon sea salt

1. Place all the ingredients in a large blender in the order listed so the liquids and the mashed banana are at the bottom.

2. Blend on high speed for 30 to 60 seconds or until the mixture is smooth, scraping down the sides as needed.

3. Let the mixture stand in the blender for 2 to 3 minutes to let the coconut flour thicken.

4. Blend again on medium speed for 30 seconds to smooth it out again. The batter will be thick.

5. Heat a large skillet over medium heat and grease the pan with coconut oil or cooking spray as desired.

6. Pour the batter out into pancakes about 5 inches in diameter. Smooth out just a bit after pouring.

7. Cook until bubbles form on the surface and the edges begin to brown, 3 to 5 minutes, then flip and cook the other side. Enjoy immediately.

NUTRITION INFORMATION PER PANCAKE
Total Protein: 9g   Collagen Protein: 5g
Calories: 154   Carbohydrates: 16g   Fat: 7g   Fiber: 3g

Blueberry Protein Pancakes

Pancakes don't have to be a guilty pleasure breakfast—with this recipe, you can feel good about getting your day off to a nutritious and delicious start! Great choice for families with children who prefer a sweet vs. savory breakfast.

Yield: 4 large pancakes | Total Time: 30 minutes

3 eggs

1 cup ricotta cheese

¼ cup collagen peptides

½ teaspoon vanilla extract

¼ cup regular or gluten-free pancake mix

½ cup frozen or fresh blueberries

1 tablespoon melted butter, ghee, or other oil

real maple syrup, for serving

1. In a medium bowl, whisk together the eggs, ricotta cheese, collagen peptides, vanilla, and pancake mix until smooth.

2. Lightly butter or oil a large skillet over medium-high heat.

3. Pour the batter into the skillet in 4-inch pancakes and immediately drop blueberries onto pancakes. Cook 3 to 5 minutes, flip, and cook 3 to 5 minutes longer.

4. Serve with real maple syrup—a little goes a long way!

NUTRITION INFORMATION PER PANCAKE
Total Protein: 18g   Collagen Protein: 7g
Calories: 250   Carbohydrates: 11g   Fat: 15g   Fiber: 1g

Coconut Collagen Coffee "Creamer"

If you're like many people, your first cup of coffee is a treasured morning ritual that mustn't be messed with. For me, only half-and-half would do to lighten my organic decaf. I didn't even want to put collagen protein in my coffee for fear it would change the taste. Enter this simple mixture of dry ingredients. I developed this blend to help patients who were not consuming dairy, but still wanted a way to add "cream" to their coffee, tea, or hot chocolate, as well as a collagen protein boost to start their day. I find that it is actually a pretty good substitute for half-and-half. This "creamer" is a snap to mix up and keeps quite well in the pantry. It also dissolves well in hot beverages.

There's an added bonus in this mix: readily absorbable calcium from bone meal powder. Almost none of my dairy-free patients get adequate amounts of calcium from their diet, despite a fairly good intake of greens and other vegetables. They are quite surprised when we review the micronutrient analysis of their diets: Most of them have calcium intakes below 500 mg per day, in contrast with the general recommendation to consume at least 800 mg or more, depending on body size.

The addition of just ¼ teaspoon of bone meal powder (I like Kal brand) per serving supplies a hefty 325 mg calcium, about one-third of the daily amount recommended—even more than an 8-ounce glass of milk! Bone meal is almost 30 percent collagen protein, but the contribution from bone meal in a 2-tablespoon serving of this creamer is fairly low, just slightly less than ½ gram of collagen.

Yield: 8 (2-tablespoon) servings | Total Time: 5 minutes

1 cup hydrolyzed collagen or collagen peptides

1 cup coconut cream powder

2 teaspoons bone meal powder

1 teaspoon vanilla extract powder or ground cinnamon (optional)

1. Mix the dry ingredients together well and store in an airtight container.

2. To serve, stir 2 tablespoons into a hot beverage.

NUTRITION INFORMATION PER SERVING
Total Protein: 5.5g   Collagen Protein: 5.5g
Calories: 110   Carbohydrates: 6g   Fat: 7g   Fiber: 1g

Guacamole

This super-easy recipe is sure to become a versatile mainstay in your diet. A small amount of collagen protein isn't noticeable at all, and I love the blend of avocado, lime, and salt—I think nothing else is needed to make a great guacamole. But you can add a few dashes of hot sauce, some chopped tomatoes, and/or minced cilantro to give it your personal touch.

Yield: 4 (½-cup) servings | Total Time: 10 minutes

2 medium ripe avocados

1 ½ tablespoons hydrolyzed collagen

juice of 1 lime (about 2 tablespoons)

1 teaspoon salt

1. Halve the avocados and scoop out the soft flesh into a medium bowl. Mash with fork.

2. Mix in the remaining ingredients and serve immediately.

3. Store any leftovers in the refrigerator with plastic wrap on the surface to prevent browning.

NUTRITION INFORMATION PER SERVING
Total Protein: 5g   Collagen Protein: 4g
Calories: 130   Carbohydrates: 7g   Fat: 11g   Fiber: 5g

Bloody Mary Aspic with Shrimp

This is a fun and easy way to serve shrimp—and hearkens back to the 1950s and '60s when savory gelatin molds were popular. I like a dark, full-flavored beer for this recipe.

Yield: 8 (¾ -cup) servings | Total Time: 60 minutes (plus 3 to 5 hours to chill)

5 tablespoons unflavored gelatin powder

3 cups tomato juice

2 tablespoons vodka

½ cup beer

1 tablespoon Worcestershire sauce

1 tablespoon lemon juice

½ teaspoon salt

1 teaspoon black pepper

3 dashes hot sauce, or to taste

1 pound shrimp, steamed in shells, peeled and diced

½ cup shrimp cooking liquid

¼ cup thinly sliced green olives

celery sticks, to garnish

1. In a small saucepan, sprinkle the gelatin evenly over the tomato juice and allow the gelatin to absorb the liquid for 2 minutes.

2. Bring tomato juice to just boiling over medium heat while whisking well until the gelatin is fully dissolved, 10 to 15 minutes.

3. Transfer the gelatin to a medium bowl and allow the mixture to cool to room temperature, 30 to 45 minutes.

4. Mix in the vodka, beer, Worcestershire sauce, lemon juice, salt, pepper, and hot sauce. Stir in the shrimp and its cooking liquid.

5. Refrigerate until slightly thickened, 1 to 2 hours, and stir in the olives.

6. Transfer the gelatin to a mold and refrigerate until firm, 2 to 3 hours. Unmold, garnish with celery sticks, and serve.

NUTRITION INFORMATION PER SERVING
Total Protein: 20g   Collagen Protein: 4
Calories: 115   Carbohydrates: 5g   Fat: 1g   Fiber: <1g

Shrimp Cocktail Mold

This is a non-alcoholic version of the Bloody Mary Aspic with Shrimp (page 164).

Yield: 4 (1-cup) servings | Total Time: 20 minutes (plus 3 to 5 hours to chill)

½ cup unflavored gelatin powder

⅓ cup room-temperature water

1 cup boiling water

2 cups tomato juice

1 tablespoon lemon juice

2 tablespoons prepared horseradish

1 cup finely chopped celery

¼ teaspoon salt

⅛ teaspoon black pepper

1 cup coarsely chopped cooked shrimp

lettuce leaves, for serving

1. Sprinkle the gelatin onto the ⅓ cup room-temperature water in a medium bowl. Allow to fully hydrate for 5 minutes.

2. Add the boiling water and stir to completely dissolve.

3. Mix in the remaining ingredients, except the lettuce, and pour into a gelatin mold or medium glass bowl.

4. Refrigerate for 3 to 5 hours until firm.

5. Cut into 2-inch squares and serve on lettuce leaves.

NUTRITION INFORMATION PER SERVING
Total Protein: 22g   Collagen Protein: 12g
Calories: 120   Carbohydrates: 7g   Fat: 1g   Fiber: 1g

"Refried" Black Bean Dip

Serve this dip with tortilla chips, raw vegetables, or as a side dish to any Mexican-style meal. The collagen protein and cheese substantially increase the protein content and quality of this and any other dried bean dish you make. I like to use grass-fed New Zealand cheddar in this recipe.

Yield: 4 (½-cup) servings | Total Time: 20 minutes

1 tablespoon olive oil, or bacon fat or lard, if desired

¼ cup chopped fresh green chiles or 1 (4.5-ounce) can chopped green chiles

2 cloves garlic, minced

2 cups cooked black turtle beans, drained

½ teaspoon salt

juice of ½ lime

2 rounded tablespoons collagen peptides

4 ounces sharp cheddar cheese, shredded

2 tablespoons minced cilantro (optional)

1. Warm the olive oil or other fat in a large frying pan over medium heat. Add the chiles and cook for 3 to 5 minutes until soft, then add the garlic and cook for 1 minute more. If using canned chiles, cook the garlic first and then add the chiles when you add the beans.

2. Mix in the beans and salt and cook for another few minutes to blend the flavors.

3. Transfer to a food processor, add the lime juice and collagen peptides, then process until smooth, 3 to 5 minutes. There will be some specks of black bean skins visible throughout, and this is normal.

4. To serve, reheat in a pan or in the microwave, then top with shredded cheese and cilantro, if using.

NUTRITION INFORMATION PER SERVING

Total Protein: 18g   Collagen Protein: 4g

Calories: 290   Carbohydrates: 22g   Fat: 44g   Fiber: 8g

Poultry Bone Broth

Good bone broth supplies more than just collagen and some minerals. It also contains type II joint collagen, glycosaminoglycans like hyaluronic acid, and chondroitin sulfate.

If you want to eat the meat in the final soup, make sure you remove it from the broth after 1 to 2 hours because if it cooks much longer, the texture and flavor may not be appealing.

Yield: 2 to 3 quarts | Total Time: 4 to 12 hours

1 tablespoon olive oil, or duck fat or ghee

6 to 8 whole chicken wings

carcass from a roast chicken, including the meat that clings to the bones and skin

water

1. Heat the olive oil or other fat in a large, heavy pot over medium-high heat, then brown the chicken wings.

2. Add the chicken carcass and all its pieces, and enough water to cover.

3. Slowly bring to a boil over medium heat, then reduce the heat to a simmer. Do not cover, but make sure to top off with additional water to keep bones covered.

4. Allow to simmer for at least 4 hours, or up to 12 hours for a deeper flavor.

5. Freeze extra broth immediately after cooling if you don't plan on using it in 5 to 7 days.

NUTRITION INFORMATION PER CUP
Total Protein: 5.5g   Collagen Protein: 5.5g
Calories: 110   Carbohydrates: 6g   Fat: 7g   Fiber: 0g

MAKING THE BEST POULTRY BONE BROTH

1. Start with the best chicken or turkey you can buy; this is the most important factor in the flavor. The tastiest broth I ever made started with older chickens called "spent layers" by the Amish farmer that sold them. Pasture-raised chicken is also very good, followed by organic chicken.

2. See if you can get some chicken feet, necks, or extra wings to up the collagen content.

3. If you have time, roast or brown the chicken parts first to achieve a slightly deeper-colored and richer broth. Or use the leftovers from a roasted bird; just make sure you keep a good deal of the skin and some of the meat that clings to the bones for flavor in the broth.

4. During cooking, keep the bones covered with water at all times, but don't add a lot of extra water—the broth may become too weak. (I also like to cover the pot so it does not lose too much liquid, but this is optional, especially if you want to slowly concentrate the stock.)

5. To make a clearer broth, drag a fine-mesh strainer several times through the finished liquid, after removing the larger pieces of bone, etc. You can also pour the broth through a strainer into another large pot.

Beef Bone Broth

There is no substitute for a good homemade broth, and it's a snap to make. Bones from pastured livestock generally produce tastier broths than standard supermarket bones. A mixture of marrow, joint, and meatier bones will yield the richest flavor, as will browning the bones before adding water.

For the best result, it is important to use cold water to start and maintain a slow simmer, otherwise you can end up with a cloudy stock. Avoid covering the pot, as this will lead to a too-rapid boil. The resulting evaporation dries out the surface scum, making it easier to skim off.

I generally like a very plain bone broth—this has the most versatility in recipes. I use the broth to cook grains like rice and barley, and to add to a variety of gravies and sauces. Bone broth is a fair source of minerals, with approximately 100 milligrams of calcium per quart.

Yield: 16 (1-cup) servings | Total Time: 6 to 12 hours

4 pounds beef marrow and joint bones

2 to 3 pounds meaty rib or neck bones

1 tablespoon olive oil or other fat

½ cup apple cider vinegar (optional)

4 to 6 cups chopped onions, celery, and carrots, or other root vegetables (optional)

2 cloves garlic, chopped (optional)

1 teaspoon dried herbs (optional)

2 bay leaves (optional)

salt and pepper, to taste (optional)

1. Preheat oven to 400°F. In a large roasting pan or heavy stock pot, roast the raw bones until medium brown, 20 to 30 minutes. Turn bones halfway through to ensure an even color. If you prefer a lighter colored broth, cover the bones with water in the stock pot, bring to a boil, and discard the water, then skip to step 4.

2. Cool the bones in the pot or pan for 15 minutes, then pour off and discard any fat that has accumulated, taking care not to pour off browned bits and juices.

3. If using a roasting pan, transfer the bones to a heavy stock pot. To transfer the flavorful bits of browned juices, mix in a cup of water, stir to loosen, and pour into the stock pot.

4. Add cold water to cover plus 2 inches to the pot, and stir to loosen any bits on bottom of pot. Add vinegar now if desired.

5. Bring to a gentle simmer on low heat and simmer for 4 to 10 hours. Do not cover. Add more water if level drops below the bones.

6. Periodically, skim off the scum that collects on the surface and discard.

7. In the last 2 hours of cooking, add any optional ingredients.

8. Remove the bone broth from the heat. After cooling slightly, pour broth through a strainer into a second larger pot. Discard the bones and vegetables.

9. Excess fat can be skimmed off hot broth by adding ice cubes, which cause the fat to slightly congeal for easier removal. Alternatively, you can remove the fat after cooling, or leave fat on the top of the storage container to keep the broth fresher. I generally transfer to quart-size mason jars after the broth has cooled for 1 hour. These can be stored in the refrigerator for one week. If you wish to freeze the broth to keep for a few months, transfer after refrigeration to appropriate plastic containers.

NUTRITION INFORMATION PER SERVING
Total Protein: 6g   Collagen Protein: 5g
Calories: 35   Carbohydrates: 2g   Fat: <1g   Fiber: 0g

Easy Chicken Soup

When you don't have any bone broth lying around, shelf-stable gelatin or collagen peptides can come in handy to make a nourishing soup. Using canned or boxed chicken stock for part of the water will intensify the flavor.

Yield: 6 (2-cup) servings | Total Time: 45 minutes

6 cups water (or 3 cups water and 3 cups chicken stock)

1 pound boneless chicken breasts or thighs, skin-on

2 tablespoons olive oil

2 large carrots, peeled and chopped

1 large onion, chopped

4 celery ribs, chopped

1 pound potatoes, peeled and cubed

2 cups raw spinach leaves

1 teaspoon sea salt

1 teaspoon black pepper

¼ cup unflavored gelatin powder or collagen peptides

1. Heat the water (or water and chicken stock) in a large pot over medium-high heat until boiling.

2. Add the chicken and cover the pot. Cook until the chicken is cooked through, 15 to 20 minutes.

3. Skim any foam off the top of the water. Remove the chicken and set aside. Once cooled, cube or chop the chicken into chunks. Discard the skin if desired. Reserve the cooking water.

4. Warm the olive oil in a second large pot over medium heat. Add the carrots, onion, and celery, and cook until translucent, 5 to 10 minutes.

5. Add the potatoes and the reserved cooking water. Bring the water to a simmer and cook until the potatoes are tender, about 15 minutes.

6. Turn the heat off. Stir in the chicken, spinach, salt, and pepper. Stir in the gelatin or collagen peptides.

NUTRITION INFORMATION PER SERVING
Total Protein: 30.6g   Collagen Protein: 4.6g
Calories: 284   Carbohydrates: 21.9g   Fat: 8g   Fiber: 3.5g

Italian Wedding Soup

Prepare the meatballs from the recipe on page 192, but form them into 1-inch balls for this soup. If you're avoiding gluten, short-grain rice is a good substitute for the pasta.

Yield: 6 (2-cup) servings | Total Time: 30 minutes

1 tablespoon extra-virgin olive oil

2 or 3 cloves garlic, minced (about 1 tablespoon)

2 quarts Poultry Bone Broth (page 169)

2 tablespoons unflavored gelatin powder

½ cup cool water

¾ cup small dried pasta, such as acini de pepe

cooked Italian Meatballs (page 192)

8 ounces fresh baby spinach

salt and black pepper

grated Parmesan cheese, for serving

1. Heat the olive oil in a large pot over medium-high heat. Add the garlic and sauté for 3 minutes.

2. Add the broth and bring to a boil.

3. In the meantime, stir gelatin into water and allow to fully hydrate.

4. Add the pasta, return to a boil, then reduce the heat and simmer for 10 minutes, until al dente, or just slightly firm.

5. Add the meatballs and gelatin and simmer 5 minutes more, until the meatballs are heated through.

6. Stir in the spinach and immediately turn off the heat. Let sit for 10 minutes before serving to allow the spinach to wilt.

7. Season with salt and pepper to taste, sprinkle with Parmesan cheese.

NUTRITION INFORMATION PER SERVING

Total Protein: 28g   Collagen Protein: 2.3g

Calories: 390   Carbohydrates: 23g   Fat: 21g   Fiber: 3g

Cream of Vegetable Soup

This is a great way to incorporate more seasonal vegetables into your diet and use up those assorted leftover vegetables. I like asparagus, zucchini, broccoli, and spinach for a green spring and summer soup; and butternut squash, parsnips, and carrots for an orange fall and winter soup. Herbs for the green soup include chives, flat-leaf parsley, basil, and savory, while spices for the orange soup are nutmeg, cardamom, ginger, and pumpkin pie spice. The potato is added to thicken the soup; use a white potato for the green soup, and a sweet potato for the orange soup.

Yield: 6 (2-cup) servings | Total Time: 30 minutes

1 tablespoon butter

½ cup chopped white onion

1 teaspoon preferred spice or spice blend or 2 tablespoons chopped fresh herbs

2 quarts Poultry Bone Broth (page 169) or prepared chicken stock

4 tablespoons unflavored gelatin powder dissolved in ½ cup cool water *or* 4 tablespoons collagen peptides (if using chicken stock)

1 large white or sweet potato, peeled and sliced into ½-inch slices

3 cups sliced or chopped raw vegetables

½ cup sour or heavy cream

salt and black pepper

1. In a heavy 6-quart pot, melt the butter over medium heat and sauté the onion until translucent, but without browning, about 10 minutes.

2. Add the spices, if using, and cook 1 minute longer. If using herbs, reserve until the end so as not to overcook.

3. Add the poultry bone broth or chicken stock (if using chicken stock, and fortifying with gelatin, first dissolve the gelatin in ½ cup cool water and then add to pot. If fortifying with collagen protein, you can add directly to pot). Bring to a boil over medium heat.

4. Add the potato, return to a low boil over medium heat, and cook until the potato is almost tender, about 10 minutes.

5. Add the vegetables, return to low boil, and cook until just tender. If making a green soup, you want your vegetables to retain some of their bright green color but still be tender, so be careful not to overcook. Spinach and other tender greens should be added last as they need only 2 to 3 minutes to cook.

6. Turn off heat. With handheld blender, puree until smooth. You can also transfer to a traditional blender, but you may want to allow the soup to cool first to avoid spattering hot liquid.

7. Whisk in the sour or heavy cream, and season with salt and pepper to taste.

8. If using fresh herbs, sprinkle on top of each bowl.

NUTRITION INFORMATION PER SERVING
Total Protein: 18g   Collagen Protein: 4g
Calories: 245   Carbohydrates: 25g   Fat: 10g   Fiber: 3g

Salmon Skin Salad

Ask your fish monger to remove the skin for you. You can use the remainder of the salmon for your main course.

Yield: 4 (1¼-cup) servings | Total Time: 20 minutes

skin of ½ pound salmon fillets

4 cups spring mix (baby lettuce mix of greens, lettuces, and radicchio)

½ cup thinly sliced English cucumbers, peeled if desired

½ cup grape tomatoes, halved

handful of mung bean or daikon sprouts

thinly sliced green onions (optional)

generous pinch of katsuobushi (dried bonito fish shavings), for garnish (optional)

toasted sesame seeds, for garnish (optional)

Japanese ponzu or equal parts freshly squeezed lemon juice and soy sauce

toasted sesame oil

1. Using a sharp knife, slice the salmon skin into thin strips. Alternatively, use kitchen shears. If there is any flesh or fat attached to the salmon skin, leave this on, as it will add flavor to the salad.

2. Grill the salmon skin: Line a baking sheet with foil and spray lightly with cooking spray. Place the strips of salmon skin on the foil. Preheat the oven's broiler (or use a toaster oven). Broil the salmon skin until the skin is browned or slightly crisp, 3 to 4 minutes. (Be very careful, as it burns easily if you don't watch it!)

3. Divide the spring mix into four small bowls.

4. Top the greens with cucumbers, tomatoes, and sprouts. Add the green onions, if desired.

5. Top the salad with the crisp salmon skin pieces.

6. Garnish with katsuobushi or toasted sesame seeds, if desired.

7. Serve with ponzu sauce and toasted sesame oil, or another Asian-style dressing.

NUTRITION INFORMATION PER SERVING
Total Protein: 7.5g   Collagen Protein: 6g
Calories: 235   Carbohydrates: 23g   Fat: 15g   Fiber: 4g

Lemon Tahini Salad Dressing and Dip

You love to eat a healthy salad, but sometimes wonder if adding dressing could be undoing all the good you are doing for yourself. Good news: This dressing actually increases the healthfulness of your salad! It's loaded with tahini, a "butter" made from sesame seeds, one of the best sources of a full-spectrum of vitamin E. (Did you know there are actually eight kinds of vitamin E?)

Say sayonara to fat-free dips and dressings—you need the fat to best absorb those supernutrients: the carotenoids, lutein, and zeaxanthin in the colorful vegetables. Even better, the lemon juice is alkalizing for the body, and the raw garlic, well, what isn't raw garlic good for? And as an added bonus, you get 3 grams of collagen protein in just 2 tablespoons of dressing. You won't even notice it, but your body definitely will!

If you find this dressing a bit too lemony, just increase the tahini by 2 tablespoons and/or add an additional ⅛ teaspoon salt. Because it is fairly thick, it is great for dipping raw veggies or perhaps crackers or even falafel balls. If you like a thinner dressing, just add a bit of water.

Yield: 5 ounces (10 tablespoons) | Total Time: 15 minutes (plus 2 hours to thicken)

¼ cup tahini

juice of 1 lemon (about ⅓ cup)

1 or 2 whole cloves garlic

¼ teaspoon salt

2 tablespoons collagen peptides, stirred into ¼ cup warm water

few dashes ground cumin (optional)

Blend all of the ingredients in a blender or food processor, and refrigerate for 2 hours to thicken before serving.

NUTRITION INFORMATION PER OUNCE
Total Protein: 6g   Collagen Protein: 3g
Calories: 90   Carbohydrates: 4g   Fat: 6g   Fiber: 2g

Lentil-Parsley Salad

I love lentils when they are prepared well. My favorite way is in a cold, Mediterranean-style salad, and this one is slightly tart and very refreshing. It's loaded with almost 20 grams of protein and 500 mg of potassium, 25 and 10 percent of your daily needs, respectively. And lentils are one of the best dietary sources of folate and fiber, along with minerals like magnesium. Plus, parsley is a superfood—one of the highest-antioxidant greens we can eat.

The best way to prepare lentils is to soak them in water overnight, then drain them before cooking. You will both cut the total cooking time by one-third and enhance their digestibility too if you pre-soak. You can also find sprouted lentils in some natural grocery stores; these have been pre-sprouted and dried and don't need to be soaked in advance.

Yield: 8 (⅔-cup) servings | Total Time: 3½ hours (including cooking and cooling)

2 cups lentils

3 cloves garlic, minced

4 tablespoons olive oil, divided

2 cups chicken bone broth

¼ cup hydrolyzed collagen

¼ cup lemon juice, from about 1 medium lemon

1 teaspoon salt

¼ teaspoon black pepper

2 medium tomatoes, coarsely chopped

½ cup chopped flat-leaf parsley, loosely packed

1. Rinse the lentils and place in a medium bowl. Cover with cool water by 2 inches and allow to soak overnight or all day at room temperature.

2. When the lentils have finished soaking and you are ready to prepare salad, start by mincing garlic cloves and allowing to sit for 10 minutes to fully develop their antioxidant potential.

3. Put 2 tablespoons of the olive oil into medium sauce pan over medium heat. Add the garlic and sauté for 2 to 3 minutes, until softened.

4. Drain the lentils and add to the pan along with the bone broth. Bring to a boil and simmer for about 1 hour, or until tender. You may need to add water; do not let the lentils become dry.

5. Remove from the heat and allow to cool for 30 minutes at room temperature.

6. Sprinkle the collagen on top of lentils and stir into the warm mixture.

7. Transfer the lentil mixture into a bowl and refrigerate for 1 to 2 hours, until cold.

8. Stir in the remaining 2 tablespoons olive oil and the lemon juice, salt, and pepper.

9. Fold in tomatoes and parsley, and serve immediately or refrigerate until serving.

NUTRITION INFORMATION PER SERVING
Total Protein: 19g   Collagen Protein: 6g
Calories: 260   Carbohydrates: 34g   Fat: 8g   Fiber: 6g

Mashed Potatoes

You probably think of mashed potatoes as a comfort food that doesn't have a lot of nutritional benefit. But before you dismiss the lowly potato, did you know that it's one of the best dietary sources of potassium and contains a fair amount of protein all on its own? Could mashed potatoes be made better with the addition of collagen protein? Absolutely!

Yield: 8 (⅔-cup) servings | Total Time: 45 minutes

8 to 10 medium russet potatoes, peeled (about 2 pounds)

5 tablespoons collagen peptides

½ cup chicken bone broth, at room temperature

2 tablespoons butter

1 teaspoon salt

¼ teaspoon black pepper

1. Place the potatoes in a large pot, cover with water, and boil until soft, 30 to 45 minutes, depending on the size of the potatoes. Do not cut the potatoes into small pieces to speed cooking, as a lot of valuable potassium is leached into the water that way.

2. Pour off the cooking water and mash the potatoes with potato masher.

3. Dissolve the collagen protein in the bone broth.

4. Add the bone broth, butter, salt, and pepper to potatoes, and stir well.

NUTRITION INFORMATION PER SERVING
Total Protein: 8g   Collagen Protein: 5.5g
Calories: 175   Carbohydrates: 22g   Fat: 7g   Fiber: 8g

Roasted Vegetables

You can roast almost any vegetable using this recipe, but my favorites are zucchini, butternut squash, green and red peppers, cauliflower, parsnips, carrots, onions, and brussels sprouts. If you do a vegetable medley, make sure you cut the firmer vegetables somewhat smaller than the softer vegetables to ensure even cooking times.

Yield: 4 (1-cup) servings | Total Time: 1 hour

6 cups chopped vegetables of choice

2 tablespoons red wine vinegar

2 tablespoons olive oil

¼ cup collagen peptides

2 teaspoons dried rosemary or other herb

sea salt and black pepper, to taste

1. Preheat the oven to 425°F.

2. Arrange the vegetables on a large baking sheet. In a small bowl, combine the red wine vinegar, olive oil, collagen peptides, and dried rosemary. Whisk well until the peptides are dissolved. Pour over the vegetables and toss to coat.

3. Bake for 20 minutes, then remove the pan to toss the vegetables.

4. Bake another 20 minutes, or until the vegetables begin to turn golden and soften.

5. Serve the vegetables with the sauce created in the pan and top with sea salt and pepper to taste.

NUTRITION INFORMATION PER SERVING
Total Protein: 9g   Collagen Protein: 7g
Calories: 123   Carbohydrates: 7g   Fat: 7g   Fiber: 3–5g

Ginger Chicken Curry

This is a very easy recipe that is absolutely delicious. You can use boneless chicken thighs if you prefer; removing the skin from the chicken is optional.

Yield: 4 (1¼-cup) servings | Total Time: 45 minutes (plus 2 to 8 hours for marinating)

2 tablespoons minced fresh ginger

2 tablespoons minced garlic

1 tablespoon red curry paste

1 bunch cilantro, chopped, divided

juice of 1 lime

2 tablespoons olive oil, divided

1 pound boneless chicken breasts, cut into 1-inch chunks

2 medium white onions, diced

1 teaspoon ground turmeric

1 (15-ounce) can full-fat coconut milk

¼ cup collagen peptides

½ teaspoon sea salt

1. In a large bowl, combine the ginger, garlic, curry paste, half of the chopped cilantro, lime juice, and 1 tablespoon of the olive oil until a paste forms.

2. Combine with chicken breast chunks and marinate in the refrigerator for at least 2 hours and up to 8 hours.

3. Heat the remaining 1 tablespoon of olive oil over medium-high heat in a large saucepan.

4. Add the onions and sauté for about 6 minutes, until soft. Add the turmeric and cook for another minute.

5. Add the marinated chicken to the pan and cook for 5 minutes, until the outside of the chicken is cooked.

6. Add the coconut milk, collagen peptides, and sea salt. Cover and let simmer for 30 minutes, until the chicken is cooked through and the flavors meld together.

7. Stir in the remaining cilantro and serve.

NUTRITION INFORMATION PER SERVING
Total Protein: 43g   Collagen Protein: 7g
Calories: 363   Carbohydrates: 14g   Fat: 15g   Fiber: 1.5g

Sesame-Glazed Chicken Wings

This is just one way to prepare chicken wings, which are a great way to get more collagen protein in your diet because they have a high ratio of skin to meat. Chicken wings are great for kids, especially the meatier or "drumette" pieces, which are easy for even small children to hold and eat. Time to change it up from the chicken nuggets!

Yield: 4 (3-wing) servings | Total Time: 45 minutes

½ cup low-sodium soy sauce

2-inch piece fresh ginger, peeled and minced

5 garlic cloves, minced

2 fresh red chiles, minced, or 1 tablespoon red pepper sauce

2 pounds chicken wings (about 12 wings)

⅓ cup ketchup

⅓ cup rice wine vinegar

3 tablespoons honey or corn syrup

¼ cup hulled sesame seeds

3 green onions, finely sliced

1. In a medium bowl, combine the soy sauce, ginger, garlic, and chiles or red pepper sauce.

2. Add chicken wings and let marinate for 15 minutes, stirring often, poking with a fork to help the marinade penetrate.

3. Preheat the oven to 425°F (on convection bake or roast if that is available). Place wings on a foil-lined baking or cookie sheet, or if preferred, on a lightly oiled slotted roasting rack. Roast wings 10 minutes, then turn and roast an additional 5 to 10 minutes. The wings should just begin to look golden brown before turning.

4. While the wings are roasting, in a small bowl, combine the ketchup, rice wine vinegar, and honey or corn syrup.

5. Increase the oven temperature to 450°F. Using a basting brush, coat the chicken wings with half of the ketchup mixture. Roast 5 to 10 minutes longer.

6. Turn chicken wings once more, coat with the remaining ketchup mixture, and generously sprinkle with sesame seeds. Roast 5 to 10 more minutes until the seeds are slightly toasted.

7. Transfer to a platter. Sprinkle with thinly sliced green onions and serve.

NUTRITION INFORMATION PER SERVING
Total Protein: 26g   Collagen Protein: No data
Calories: 415   Carbohydrates: 30g   Fat: 22g   Fiber: 1g

Beef Stew

A good-old fashioned meal is made even better with collagen protein and Brussels sprouts. If you can make your own homemade bone broth from grass-fed beef bones, so much the better. But if you're like me and have difficulty finding the time to make everything from scratch (not to mention finding a source for the bones!), keeping a few boxes of ready-made bone broth in the pantry is the answer; I like the Kettle and Fire brand, but there are other quality products. This stew uses mashed potatoes as thickener, which is great if you are avoiding wheat or gluten! If you don't have potatoes available, 2 to 3 tablespoons of flour thickens equally well. As written, this recipe is happily gluten- and dairy-free.

Yield: 4 (2¼-cup) servings | Total Time: 3½ hours (up to 8 if using a slow cooker)

1 tablespoon olive oil

1 pound stew beef cubes

3 cups bone broth, preferably beef flavor

1½ cups coarsely chopped white onion

3 medium carrots, peeled and sliced into ½-inch rounds

1 teaspoon dried thyme

1 teaspoon salt

¼ teaspoon black pepper

1 pound fresh Brussels sprouts, ends and wilted outer leaves removed

¼ cup collagen peptides

1 cup prepared mashed potatoes

1. In a large, heavy saucepan, warm the olive oil over medium-high heat for 1 minute. .

2. Add the beef cubes and brown lightly on all sides.

3. Add the bone broth and simmer for 2 to 3 hours, or until the beef is almost tender. You can also transfer everything to a slow cooker for 6 to 8 hours on medium heat.

4. Add the onion, carrots, thyme, salt, and pepper to the stew, and cook 15 more minutes.

5. Add the brussels sprouts and cook an additional 10 minutes.

6. Turn off the heat, sprinkle the collagen on the top surface, and stir into the stew.

7. Stir in the mashed potatoes to thicken the stew before serving.

NUTRITION INFORMATION PER SERVING
Total Protein: 38g   Collagen Protein: 12g
Calories: 420   Carbohydrates: 34g   Fat: 17g   Fiber: 7g

Italian Meatballs

I almost never miss an opportunity to try a meatball when I eat at a fine Italian restaurant. To me, the ideal meatball is plump, moist, and fine-textured with a blend of flavors—garlic, cheese, herbs, and of course, meat! I prefer meatballs with garlic but no onion; if you wish to add minced onion to this recipe, you can do so to your taste—half a cup is probably a good place to start.

For the meat, I like to use grass-fed beef. If you're avoiding pork, all beef is fine. And the bacon is optional, but it can help make for a moister meatball, especially if the beef is less than 20 percent fat. You may choose to finely chop the beef and pork with a couple of chef's knives on a larger cutting board. This is an optional step, especially if you get finely ground meat from your butcher. I don't like to have my meat ground again in the store (more bacterial contamination risk) but that is another option. The finer the grind of the meat, the finer the texture of the meatball.

While this recipe is neither gluten- nor dairy-free, a couple easy swaps will get you there: Use an extra ⅓ cup bone broth in place of the buttermilk and ½ cup finely chopped cooked mushrooms in place of the Parmesan if you're avoiding dairy. I like to make my own gluten-free bread crumbs in the food processor from oven-dried gluten-free bread.

Yield: 8 (2-ounce) meatballs | Total Time: 90 minutes

½ cup bone broth, or beef or chicken stock, at room temperature

2 tablespoons unflavored gelatin powder

⅓ cup buttermilk (or ¼ cup plain yogurt with water added to make ⅓ cup)

1 cup dried plain bread crumbs

1 pound ground beef

1 pound ground pork

4 teaspoons fresh garlic, finely chopped

½ cup grated Parmesan cheese

3 slices thick-cut bacon, chopped

2 teaspoons sea salt

2 large eggs plus 2 egg yolks

2 teaspoons Italian seasoning

2 tablespoons finely minced flat-leaf parsley

1. Pour the broth or stock into a microwaveable cup and sprinkle the gelatin on top. Allow to sit for 5 minutes so the gelatin absorbs the liquid, then microwave for 90 seconds to dissolve. Stir the mixture and place the cup in ice water or in the refrigerator until gelatin firms up, 15 to 30 minutes. Once firm, slice into small pieces without removing from the cup. This will be added to the meat mixture as the last ingredient.

2. Preheat the oven to 425°F and grease a heavy casserole dish or oven-safe skillet with olive oil.

3. In a large bowl, stir the buttermilk into the bread crumbs and let sit for 5 minutes so the crumbs absorb the liquid. Break up the crumbs with a fork so there are no large clumps.

4. Mix the meats and all remaining ingredients into the bread crumbs, using your hands or a strong wooden spoon, distributing the ingredients well. Finally, mix in the pieces of gelled stock. Form the meat mixture into packed balls about 3 inches in diameter, or smaller if you wish. The gelatin pieces will be poking out a bit; try to push them into the centers of the balls.

5. Place the meatballs in the prepared baking dish and bake for 20 to 30 minutes, depending on the size of the meatballs. To test for doneness, insert a meat thermometer into the center of a meatball; it should register 150°F. I use a convection roast setting on my oven, which will speed up the cook time. You will see some juices in the pan when they are finished cooking. Don't discard them! You can add these juices to your favorite tomato sauce or use them to flavor rice or pasta, or even a soup.

This also makes a delicious meatloaf, but bake at 375°F for at least 1 hour. I like to use a Bundt pan to make meatloaf as this helps the center cook without overcooking the outside.

NUTRITION INFORMATION PER MEATBALL
Total Protein: 24g   Collagen Protein: 3g
Calories: 360   Carbohydrates: 11g   Fat: 21g   Fiber: <1g

Creole Cod

Don't like codfish or find it flavorless unless battered and fried? While authentic English pub fish and chips really does float the flavor boat, I found cooking with cod at home rather dull. Enter this easy one-pan meal: The recipe is a breeze but zings with flavor. The secret ingredients are the smoked paprika and the fermented fish sauce. My husband often wonders if I added bacon or andouille sausage when I use smoked paprika, but no! I was introduced to the versatility of fermented fish sauce while at a conference at Oxford University on the subject of Roman seafood in antiquity. Fish sauce enhances the taste of almost any food, and its "fishy" taste and smell largely dissipate after heating, leaving behind flavor and nutrients. Remember to go easy on salt if using the fish sauce; you may not need any at all.

Yield: 4 (4-ounce) servings | Total Time: 45 minutes

1 pound frozen or fresh Icelandic or other cod fillets

2 tablespoons extra-virgin olive oil

1 medium white onion, coarsely chopped

1 green bell pepper, coarsely chopped

2 to 3 cloves garlic, minced (about 1 tablespoon)

10 to 12 okra pods, halved

1 (16-ounce) can tomatoes, cut into pieces, with liquid

¾ teaspoon smoked paprika

2 bay leaves, crumbled

2 to 3 teaspoons fermented fish sauce

½ teaspoon salt, or to taste

few dashes of hot red pepper sauce, or to taste

¼ cup collagen peptides

hot, freshly cooked rice, for serving

1. Partially thaw the cod fillets if using frozen (all day in the refrigerator is best). Cut into 2-inch pieces. Set aside.

2. Heat the olive oil in large skillet over medium-high heat. Add the onion and sauté for 3 minutes.

3. Add the green pepper and garlic, and sauté for 5 more minutes.

4. Add the okra, tomatoes, smoked paprika, and bay leaves. Cover and simmer on low heat, 10 to 15 minutes. Add water as needed just to cover ingredients if the tomatoes you are using do not have a lot of liquid.

5. Gently stir in the cod, return to a simmer, and cook 5 to 10 minutes on low heat, until the fish looks firm and begins to flake, taking care not to overcook.

6. Stir in the fish sauce, salt, hot sauce, and collagen peptides, and heat 1 minute more. Serve over hot rice.

NUTRITION INFORMATION PER SERVING
Total Protein: 35g   Collagen Protein: 7g
Calories: 252   Carbohydrates: 10g   Fat: 8g   Fiber: 3g

Simple Pan-Seared Salmon

Most people do not eat the skin when they eat salmon, which is a shame as it's very nutritious and a great source of collagen protein! To get the most collagen protein-to-muscle ratio, ask the fish market to cut 4- to 6-ounce tail sections from the salmon fillets. I've found this not to be a problem at full-service grocery stores, as most shoppers want the thicker cuts toward the head of the fish anyway. Coriander is optional in this recipe; I just like the way it tastes on salmon. If you have never tried salmon with the crispy skin, I think you are in for a treat!

Yield: 4 (5-ounce) servings | Total Time: 25 minutes

4 (4- to 6-ounce) skin-on salmon filets, preferably cut from the tail end of the salmon

1 teaspoon coarse salt

½ teaspoon coarsely ground black pepper

½ teaspoon ground coriander (optional)

1 to 2 tablespoons peanut or grapeseed oil, or ghee

1. Inspect the salmon skin to make sure all the scales have been removed. To be sure, drag a knife edge crosswise against the grain of the skin to pop off any remaining scales.

2. Firmly blot the salmon fillets with paper towels to remove excess moisture. Season on both sides with salt and pepper, and season the flesh with coriander, if using. Allow to sit for 5 to 10 minutes.

3. In a large cast-iron or other heavy skillet (do not use a nonstick pan), heat the oil or ghee over medium-high heat until shimmering. Reduce the heat to medium-low, then place a salmon fillet skin-side down on the skillet.

4. Press firmly in place for 10 seconds, using the back of a large spatula, to prevent the skin from buckling. Add the remaining fillets one at a time, pressing down on each for 10 seconds.

5. Continue to sear, pressing gently on the fillets occasionally to ensure good contact with the pan, until the skin releases easily from surface of skillet, about 4 minutes. If the skin sticks to the pan when trying to lift a corner with the spatula, allow it to continue to cook until it lifts off readily.

6. Continue to cook until salmon flesh begins to firm up and lose its translucency, 10 to 15 minutes total.

7. Using spatula and a fork if needed, flip the fillets and cook on the second side for 30 seconds. Remove in same manner and serve immediately.

NUTRITION INFORMATION PER SERVING
Total Protein: 30g   Collagen Protein: No data
Calories: 245   Carbohydrates: 0g   Fiber: 0g   Fat: 13g

Baked Falafel

In my college days as a vegetarian, I used to be a "falafel fanatic." I loved the taste and thought falafel on pita bread with lettuce, tomatoes, and tahini sauce made a super-healthy lunch. Then I realized how much oil they absorbed and how unhealthy commercial frying oils were, so I stopped eating them. I still think they're delicious and make a great meal or snack, so I developed an easy, nutritious recipe for falafel that are brushed with olive oil and baked to avoid all the health issues associated with deep-frying. The addition of hydrolyzed collagen gives them a protein boost.

Please note that the recipe calls for soaked dried chickpeas—do not substitute canned or pre-cooked chickpeas or the result will not be the same. Also be aware that gluten-free flour does not work well in this recipe. For the cumin, its flavor is more robust if it is heated in 1 tablespoon olive oil for 1 to 2 minutes before adding to the falafel. Serve with Lemon Tahini Salad Dressing and Dip (page 181), lettuce, tomato, olives, and thinly sliced red onion in pita pockets.

Yield: 6 (3-falafel) servings | Total Time: 45 minutes, plus time to soak

1 cup dried chickpeas

3 tablespoons lemon juice

4 cloves garlic

1 teaspoon ground cumin

1 ½ teaspoons salt

½ teaspoon black pepper

¼ teaspoon cayenne pepper or a few dashes of red pepper sauce

6 tablespoons sesame seeds

½ bunch flat-leaf parsley

6 tablespoons collagen peptides

1 teaspoon baking powder

2 to 3 tablespoons unbleached wheat flour

¼ cup olive oil, for brushing

1. One day before cooking: Rinse the chickpeas, put into a large bowl, and cover with water plus 2 inches, as they will expand. Let soak overnight at room temperature.

2. The day of cooking, preheat the oven to 425°F and grease an insulated cookie sheet with oil, or line a regular cookie sheet with parchment paper and oil the paper.

3. Drain the chickpeas well, then put into the bowl of food processor with the remaining ingredients, except the olive oil. Add enough flour so that the dough holds together. Pulse until well chopped and the dough begins to form a mass; it should resemble cream of wheat or farina in texture.

4. Form into 18 (1½-inch) balls, then flatten into 2½-inch discs.

5. Place the falafel on the prepared cookie sheet. Brush the top surfaces with olive oil.

6. Bake for 25 to 30 minutes, turning over and brushing with oil after 15 minutes so both sides can brown lightly. Alternatively, you can cook the falafel in a small amount of olive oil in a skillet over medium heat, turning after 10 minutes or when lightly browned and cooking an additional 10 minutes on the second side.

NUTRITION INFORMATION PER SERVING
Total Protein: 22g   Collagen Protein: 8g
Calories: 400   Carbohydrates: 49g   Fat: 14g   Fiber: 12g

Coconut Chickpea Curry

My husband gave this recipe rave reviews, and I think you'll love it, too! Serve this curry as a soup or on top of rice for a main dish. If you like, add cubed chicken to increase the protein content. Chickpeas are somewhat easier to digest than most legumes, and because of their mild nutty flavor, they tend to pick up the flavors of the other ingredients they are cooked with.

Keep in mind that if you do start with dried chickpeas, make sure they are relatively fresh so they become soft after the initial cooking. In general, you don't want to store dried chickpeas, beans, or lentils for more than one year, otherwise you may find that they retain an undesirable firmness even after several hours of cooking.

Yield: 8 (⅔-cup) servings | Total Time: 45 to 75 minutes

2 tablespoons ghee or coconut oil

1 cup coarsely chopped white onion

2 cups chicken bone broth

4 cups cooked or canned chickpeas, drained

2 tablespoons red curry paste

1 teaspoon salt

5 tablespoons coconut cream powder dissolved in ½ cup hot water

¼ cup hydrolyzed collagen

½ cup chopped fresh cilantro

fresh lime

1. In a large, heavy saucepan, melt the ghee over medium heat, then add the onion and sauté for 5 to 10 minutes, until translucent and slightly brown on the edges.

2. Add the broth, chickpeas, curry paste, and salt, reduce the heat to low, and simmer for 15 to 60 minutes. The longer you let it simmer, the more the flavor soaks into the chickpeas.

3. Add the coconut cream/water mixture and simmer another 5 minutes. Turn off the heat.

4. Add the collagen by sprinkling 1 tablespoon at a time onto top of hot mixture and stirring it in well.

5. To serve, top each portion with cilantro and squeeze of lime as desired.

NUTRITION INFORMATION PER SERVING
Total Protein: 14g   Collagen Protein: 6g
Calories: 220   Carbohydrates: 26g   Fat: 7g   Fiber: 12g

Pumpkin Seed Chocolate Collagen Protein Bars

I am always looking for healthy portable snacks that I can whip up at home. There is a plethora of protein bars on the market and while some are quite good, some contain ingredients that I generally avoid. There are only a few ready-made protein bars on the market that contain collagen protein, the Bulletproof Collagen Protein Bar and the Designs for Health Pure PaleoBar are two I have tried that are delicious. Unfortunately, they both contain high amounts of fermentable fibers, which for some people can lead to flatulence. This recipe does not contain a significant amount of those potentially problematic fibers.

Yield: 12 bars | Total Time: 30 minutes

FOR THE BARS:

1 cup raw pumpkin seeds (or mixture of seeds and nuts, as desired)

1 cup unsweetened shredded coconut

½ cup melted coconut oil

½ cup collagen peptides

¼ cup pure maple syrup

½ teaspoon salt

1 teaspoon vanilla extract

FOR THE COATING:

⅓ cup coconut oil

¼ cup unsweetened cocoa powder

¼ teaspoon salt

1 tablespoon maple syrup

¼ teaspoon vanilla extract

1. Combine the pumpkin seeds, shredded coconut, and coconut oil in food processor and process until a smooth mixture forms, 5 to 10 minutes, scraping the sides with a spatula every couple of minutes.

2. Pulse in the collagen peptides, maple syrup, salt, and vanilla.

3. Turn the mixture out onto an 8 x 8-inch square pan lined with lightly oiled parchment paper. Place in freezer for 20 minutes until firm but slightly soft to the touch.

4. In a small microwave-safe bowl, combine all the coating ingredients. Microwave for 20 seconds to warm and melt the coconut oil, then stir until smooth.

5. In the pan, cut the rectangle from the freezer into 12 bars. Spread a coating of the chocolate mixture on top of them.

6. Freeze until chocolate coating is set. Transfer to an airtight container and store in the refrigerator.

NUTRITION INFORMATION PER BAR
Total Protein: 8g   Collagen Protein: 3g
Calories: 220   Carbohydrates: 11g   Fat: 25g   Fiber: 3g

Coconut Chocolate Chia "Pudding"

Love, love, love this "pudding." Couldn't be quicker to make, and it satisfies the craving for something cool, and nutritious, plus it's gluten-free, dairy-free, egg-free, and there's no cooking required! Chia seeds keep your digestive system moving along, so to speak, due to their slippery coating and high fiber content. While they contain omega-3 fats and calcium, they are not really a great source in part because we generally don't completely digest whole chia seeds. The chocolate nibs are optional, but they do lend a nice chocolate chip–like taste.

Yield: 6 (½-cup) servings | Total Time: 10 active minutes, plus 12 hours to set

¼ cup coconut sugar or raw honey

¼ to ½ cup hot water

¼ cup chocolate nibs (optional)

1 (13.5-ounce) can full-fat coconut milk

6 tablespoons hydrolyzed collagen or collagen peptides

1 teaspoon almond or vanilla extract

pinch of salt

½ cup chia seeds

1 cup sliced fresh fruit of choice (pineapple, strawberries, raspberries, bananas)

sliced or chopped almonds, pecans, or walnuts, for topping (optional)

1. If using coconut sugar, dissolve the sugar in ½ cup hot water, and add the chocolate nibs, if using. Allow to sit 30 minutes to soften. If using honey, combine with ¼ cup water and microwave for 20 to 30 seconds with the chocolate nibs, if using, or warm on the stovetop just until hot.

2. In a medium bowl, combine the coconut milk, collagen, prepared honey or coconut sugar, almond or vanilla extract, salt, and chia seeds, and mix well. Refrigerate overnight so the chia seeds can hydrate and fully thicken the mixture.

3. Serve topped with fruit, or alternate fruit and layers of pudding for a parfait. Sprinkle with chopped or sliced nuts just before serving, if desired.

NUTRITION INFORMATION PER SERVING
Total Protein: 10g   Collagen Protein: 5g
Calories: 305   Carbohydrates: 16g   Fat: 23g   Fiber: 7g

Paleo Chocolate-Avocado Freezer Fudge

A powerhouse of super foods that will satisfy your chocolate craving.

Yield: 16 squares | Total Time: 1 hour 15 minutes

1 medium avocado

⅓ cup almond butter

⅓ cup maple syrup

½ teaspoon almond extract

½ cup unsweetened cocoa powder

½ cup collagen peptides

⅛ teaspoon salt

1. In a food processor, process all ingredients until very smooth, about 5 minutes.

2. Transfer the mixture to an 8 x 8-inch baking pan lined with oiled parchment paper. Place another sheet of oiled parchment on top and flatten to spread evenly in the pan.

3. Place the pan in freezer for at least 1 hour, until moderately firm.

4. Use the parchment paper to lift the loaf from the pan and set on a cutting board.

5. Cut the fudge into 16 squares. Store in an airtight container in the freezer.

NUTRITION INFORMATION PER SQUARE
Total Protein: 5g   Collagen Protein: 3g
Calories: 80   Carbohydrates: 8g   Fat: 5g   Fiber: 2g

Coconut Collagen "Cookies"

My husband and I are avid bicyclists and often take extended rides where a portable snack comes in handy. These gluten-free, dairy-free "cookies" are great when you need quick yet sustainable energy. We have tried lots of protein/energy bars and unfortunately find that they can cause gas and bloating because of the non-digestible types of carbohydrates they contain. Note that these treats do contain fiber, just not the kind that is likely to cause gastrointestinal problems.

These cookies are a great snack for kids as well—not too sweet but with a nice chocolate flavor. If you or your child has a nut allergy, you can substitute sunflower seed butter for the almond butter, adding in 4 tablespoons of chocolate chips as you process the mixture for the chocolate flavor.

For the banana chips, be sure to choose ones that contain coconut oil, such as the Whole Foods 365 brand.

Yield: 6 (2-cookie) servings | Total Time: 55 minutes

1 cup sweetened banana chips

½ cup cocoa almond spread or another favorite nut butter

½ cup unsweetened shredded coconut

¼ cup marine collagen peptides

1 extra-large egg white

⅛ teaspoon salt

1. Preheat the oven to 250°F.

2. In a food processor, process the banana chips into a coarse powder. Add remaining ingredients and continue to process until mixture pulls away from the sides and forms a dough.

3. Form into 12 equal-size balls, place on an insulated cookie sheet or in the cups of a muffin pan, and flatten into "cookies." Bake for 30 minutes until light golden brown. Allow to cool.

4. These cookies will keep at room temperature for a few days, but for best results, store in the refrigerator.

NUTRITION INFORMATION PER SERVING
Total Protein: 7g   Collagen Protein: 5g
Calories: 260   Carbohydrates: 21g   Fat: 17g   Fiber: 3g

Protein-Powered Coconut-Pecan "Fudge"

I admit, this is a treat, but it's a healthy one! Once I got the proportions of the ingredients right—my goal was to make this taste like a mildly sweet, nutty fudge—I could not believe how much this reminded me of a favorite candy. The natural sweetness comes from the dates and coconut, and there is absolutely no added sugar. Because this is made from both collagen and whey protein, you get the benefits of collagen and the complete protein of whey to really satisfy!

Yield: 16 balls | Total Time: 20 minutes

⅓ cup coconut oil

1 cup pecan halves

½ cup pitted dates (about 16)

½ cup peanut or almond butter

⅓ cup desiccated coconut

½ cup hydrolyzed collagen

½ cup chocolate-flavored whey protein

2 teaspoons almond or vanilla extract

⅛ teaspoon salt

1. In a food processor, process the coconut oil, pecans, dates, peanut or almond butter, and desiccated coconut until crumbly.

2. Add the collagen and whey protein, almond or vanilla extract, and salt, and process until the dough pulls away from the sides, about 3 minutes.

3. Form into 16 (1½-inch) balls. Store in the refrigerator.

NUTRITION INFORMATION PER BALL
Total Protein: 6g   Collagen Protein: 1.2g
Calories: 200   Carbohydrates: 10g   Fiber: 2g   Fat: 15g

Herbal Tea or Fruit Juice Gummies

Use whatever tea you like or find therapeutic, like matcha, rooibos, or chamomile.

Yield: 10 gummies | Total Time: 15 minutes (plus 4 hours to firm)

3 tablespoons unflavored powdered gelatin

½ cup cool water

1 cup concentrated herbal tea, made with 5 or 6 tea bags, or ½ cup unsweetened fruit juice and ½ cup water

2 tablespoons honey

1. In a small saucepan, sprinkle the gelatin onto the ½ cup water and stir in well. Let sit for 3 to 5 minutes to hydrate.

2. Add the herbal tea (or fruit concentrate and water) and heat until just boiling so the gelatin dissolves.

3. Allow to cool to room temperature and stir in the honey. This is to retain the beneficial properties of the honey if you are using raw honey. If using pasteurized honey, you can add directly into the hot liquid.

4. Pour into ice cube trays or a glass dish and refrigerate until firm, about 4 hours.

5. Cut into 1- to 2-inch squares to serve.

6. Store in the refrigerator. They will keep for up to 1 week, but since they are low in sugar they will not keep as long as premade gelatin desserts.

NUTRITION INFORMATION PER GUMMY

Total Protein: 2g   Collagen Protein: 2g
Calories: 20   Carbohydrates: 5g   Fat: 0g   Fiber: 0g

Paleo Candy Sour Gummies

Do your kids like chewy, fruity treats? Why not make your own gummies and feel good about what treats you are giving them?

Yields: 6 (2-gummy) servings | Total Time: 30 minutes (plus 2 hours to chill)

2½ cups unsweetened frozen fruit such as strawberries, peaches, and mangoes

juice of 1 lemon plus water to measure ⅔ cup liquid

pinch of salt

3½ tablespoons unflavored gelatin powder

2 to three tablespoons honey or sugar*

1. Mix the gelatin into the lemon juice and water and allow to hydrate for 3 to 5 minutes.

2. Put fruit into a medium-size saucepan and stir in the gelatin mixture and salt. Stir over medium heat until the mixture just begins to simmer and the gelatin has melted, about 10 minutes.

3. Turn off the heat and allow to cool for about 15 minutes.

4. Stir in honey or sugar until dissolved.

5. Pour the warm mixture into a blender and pulse until just smooth, about 30 seconds total. Avoid overblending, as this creates excessive air bubbles.

6. Transfer the mixture into lightly oiled silicone ice cube molds or a glass baking dish.

7. Refrigerate 2 hours before removing from the molds or cutting into squares. These will keep refrigerated for up to 1 week.

* If your child is under 1 year old, substitute the honey with sugar

NUTRITION INFORMATION PER SERVING
Total Protein: 2g   Collagen Protein: 2g
Calories: 65   Carbohydrates: 15g   Fat: 1g   Fiber: 0g

Whey-Collagen Protein Smoothie

This is a versatile recipe template—by switching up the flavor of whey protein, the frozen fruit, and the type of fat used, there are dozens of different smoothies you can create. One of the best ways to maintain optimal glutathione levels (our master antioxidant) is to consume collagen protein, rich in glycine. High-quality whey protein, rich in the amino acid cysteine, will enhance glutathione production even more.

This simple recipe combines both collagen and whey. It also has kefir, which is a fermented dairy that can aid in collagen absorption. Choose a whey protein in one of your favorite flavors—chocolate, strawberry, vanilla, or if you prefer, unflavored. If you choose unflavored, you may want to add a natural sweetener like stevia or raw honey to enhance the flavor. If you are on a weight-loss diet, this is a perfect meal to start your day. It is also great any time you need an energy boost and don't have a lot of time. Super for fueling your workouts, too!

Yield: 1 serving | Total Time: 10 minutes

1 scoop or 1 rounded tablespoon collagen peptides

1 cup chopped frozen fruit (or 1 small frozen banana)

½ cup kefir or yogurt (flavored or plain)

1 tablespoon coconut cream (or 1 tablespoon nut butter or ¼ large ripe avocado)

6 to 8 ice cubes

handful of baby spinach (optional)

1 scoop (about 3 rounded tablespoons) cold-processed, non-denatured, grass-fed whey protein (such as Proserum Whey)

1. Put all the ingredients except whey protein into a blender and blend until smooth, 3 to 5 minutes, depending on the speed of your blender.

2. Add the whey protein and blend 30 to 60 seconds longer. The short blending time protects the fragile cysteine-containing protein in the whey.

3. Drink immediately or freeze for 30 minutes to eat like a soft ice cream.

NUTRITION INFORMATION PER SERVING
Total Protein: 30g   Collagen Protein: 6g
Calories: 350   Carbohydrates: 42g   Fat: 7g   Fiber: 3g

Coconut Pineapple Smoothie

This tastes like a piña colada with the nutritional boost of collagen protein. This is a dairy-free recipe, but you can substitute a yogurt made from cow's milk.

Yield: 2 servings | Total Time: 10 minutes

1 ½ cups frozen pineapple chunks

¾ cup full-fat coconut milk

2 tablespoons honey

4 rounded tablespoons collagen peptides

6 ounces coconut yogurt or almond milk yogurt

1. Add all the ingredients to a blender and blend until smooth, 3 to 5 minutes depending on the power of your blender.

2. Drink immediately or freeze for 30 minutes to eat like a soft ice cream.

NUTRITION INFORMATION PER SERVING
Total Protein: 20g   Collagen Protein: 18g
Calories: 450   Carbohydrates: 50g   Fiber: 3g   Fat: 7g

Blueberry Collagen Smoothie

This smoothie contains no dairy but has a lot of flavor; it's also Paleo and gluten-free. It is a potassium powerhouse, a mineral that most people do not get enough of. The almond butter provides extra protein.

Yield: 1 serving | Total Time: 5 minutes

1 cup coconut water, canned or frozen

2 tablespoons collagen peptides

1 handful blueberries, frozen or fresh

1 small banana, frozen

1 tablespoon almond butter

Add all the ingredients to a blender and blend for 1 to 2 minutes, until smooth and creamy.

NUTRITION INFORMATION PER SERVING
Total Protein: 18g   Collagen Protein: 12g
Calories: 380   Carbohydrates: 60g   Fat: 10g   Fiber: 11g

Green Smoothie

This is a great recipe for those who want to get their vegetables at breakfast.

Yield: 2 servings | Total Time: 5 minutes

2 cups baby spinach

1 medium apple, cored and peeled

½ medium banana

¼ avocado

2 tablespoons collagen peptides

2 tablespoons lemon juice

1 tablespoon flax or chia seeds

1 teaspoon ground turmeric

1 cup almond milk

ice (optional)

Add all the ingredients to a blender and blend for 1 to 2 minutes, until smooth.

NUTRITION INFORMATION PER SERVING

Total Protein: 10g   Collagen Protein: 7g
Calories: 176   Carbohydrates: 25g   Fat: 6g   Fiber: 6.5g

Strawberry Collagen Smoothie

You probably can see by now that almost any smoothie recipe can be pumped up with collagen protein. But keep in mind that collagen protein on its own is not a complete protein, so when you make a dairy-free shake, you will want to have another source of protein if it is part of a meal and not a snack.

Yield: 2 servings | Total Time: 5 minutes

1 cup strawberries

½ cup frozen pineapple chunks

½ cup frozen mango chunks

1 banana

2 tablespoons collagen peptides

1 cup almond milk

Add all the ingredients to a blender and blend on low speed for 30 seconds to break up any large chunks of fruit, then on high speed for 1 minute, or until smooth.

NUTRITION INFORMATION PER SERVING
Total Protein: 9g   Collagen Protein: 7g
Calories: 175   Carbohydrates: 34g   Fat: 2g   Fiber: 5g

Conclusion

When I first tossed around the idea of writing a comprehensive book on the benefits of collagen protein, I must admit that I had only a superficial understanding of what collagen protein could offer. My level of enthusiasm was somewhere around a six on a scale from one to ten. Although the research is still in its early stages, as I discovered the incredible range of benefits collagen offers, I became more and more excited to be able to share the information. I am now super-enthusiastic—definitely a 10—about the promises it holds. I am especially grateful that I learned how collagen protein can help keep us young and healthy, as I just began my seventh decade of life. Perhaps like me, you're now thinking, is there anything that collagen protein *can't* do?

Many people feel supplements are totally unnecessary if one eats a well-balanced diet. Well, I think if this book has opened your mind to one paradigm-busting idea, it is that the common understanding of what constitutes a well-balanced diet misses the mark on a number of levels. Collagen protein is a big missing piece in most people's nutrition, even when a person follows all the "expert" dietary guidelines.

Do you need to buy a collagen protein supplement to realize all of the benefits: better skin, more comfortable joints, improved detoxification, better gut health, more results from exercise, and perhaps even lower weight, blood sugar, and risk factors for cardiovascular disease? That decision is up to you. But for me, I think I will keep consuming collagen protein, whether it be collagen peptides, chicken and fish skin and bones, bone broth, gelatin, or all of the above, on a daily basis for the rest of my life. And whenever I can, I'll enjoy that bowl of pho with lots of beef tendon!

I like to keep things fairly routine, but many of my patients, and perhaps even you, like lots of variety in their diet. Whichever you prefer, I am sure you will find more than a few nutritious recipes in the next section of the book that make it easy and enjoyable to get your daily collagen protein.

Finally, I wish you the best of health so you may continue to pursue all of your goals and dreams. And I sincerely hope and pray that the information in this book will be a blessing to you and your loved ones.

Conversion Charts

Volume

U.S.	U.S. EQUIVALENT	METRIC
1 tablespoon (3 teaspoons)	½ fluid ounce	15 ml
¼ cup	2 fluid ounces	60 ml
⅓ cup	3 fluid ounces	90 ml
½ cup	4 fluid ounces	120 ml
⅔ cup	5 fluid ounces	150 ml
¾ cup	6 fluid ounces	180 ml
1 cup	8 fluid ounces	240 ml
2 cups	16 fluid ounces	480 ml

Weight

U.S.	METRIC
½ ounce	15 grams
1 ounce	30 grams
2 ounces	60 grams
¼ pound	115 grams
⅓ pound	150 grams
½ pound	225 grams
¾ pound	350 grams
1 pound	450 grams

Temperature

FAHRENHEIT (°F)	CELSIUS (°C)	FAHRENHEIT (°F)	CELSIUS (°C)
70°F	20°C	220°F	105°C
100°F	40°C	240°F	115°C
120°F	50°C	260°F	125°C
130°F	55°C	280°F	140°C
140°F	60°C	300°F	150°C
150°F	65°C	325°F	165°C
160°F	70°C	350°F	175°C
170°F	75°C	375°F	190°C
180°F	80°C	400°F	200°C
190°F	90°C	425°F	220°C
200°F	95°C	450°F	230°C

Selected References

For a full list of references, visit www.thecollagendietplan.com.

Banai, Makoto and Nobuhiro Kawai, "New Therapeutic Strategy for Amino Acid Medicine: Glycine Improves the Quality of Sleep." *Journal of Pharmacological Sciences* 118, no. 2 (2012): 145–148. doi: 10.1254/jphs.11R04FM.

Brawley, L. et al. "Glycine Rectifies Vascular Dysfunction Induced by Dietary Protein Imbalance during Pregnancy." *Journal of Physiology* 554, pt. 2 (2003): 497–504. doi: 10.1113/jphysiol.2003.052068.

Chen, Q. et al. "Collagen Peptides Ameliorate Intestinal Epithelial Barrier Dysfunction in Immunostimulatory Caco-2 Cell Monolayers via Enhancing Tight Junctions." *Food and Function* 22, no. 8 (2017): 1144–1151. doi: 10.1039/c6fo01347c.

Chiang, Tsay-I et al. "Amelioration of Estrogen-Induced Obesity by Collagen Hydrolysate." *International Journal of Medical Sciences* 13, no. 11 (2016): 853–857. doi: 10.7150/ijms.16706.

Clark, Kristine et al. "24-Week Study on the Use of Collagen Hydrolysate as a Dietary Supplement in Athletes with Activity-Related Joint Pain." *Current Medical Research and Opinion* 24, no. 5. (2008): 1485–1496. doi: 10.1185/030079908X291967

Crowley, David et al. "Safety and Efficacy of Undenatured Type II Collagen in the Treatment of Osteoarthritis of the Knee: A Clinical Trial." *International Journal of Medical Science* 6, no. 6 (2009): 312–321. doi: 10.7150/ijms.6.312.

De Luca, Chiara et al. "Skin Antiaging and Systemic Redox Effects of Supplementation with Marine Collagen Peptides and Plant-Derived Antioxidants: A Single-Blind Case Control Clinical Study." *Oxidative Medicine and Cellular Longevity* 3 (2016): 22–29. doi: 10.1155/2016/4389410.

Dennault, A. et al. "Biological Effect of Hydrolyzed Collagen on Bone Metabolism." *Critical Reviews in Food Science and Nutrition* 57, no. 9 (2017): 1922-1937. doi: 10.1080/10408398.2015.1038377.

Gannon, Mary, Jennifer Nuttall, and Frank Nuttall, "The Metabolic Response to Ingested Glycine." *American Journal of Clinical Nutrition* 76, no. 6 (2002): 1302–1307. doi: 10.1093/ajcn/76.6.1302.

Gomez-Guillen, M.C., et al. "Functional and Bioactive Properties of Collagen and Gelatin from Alternative Sources: A Review." *Food Hydrocolloids* 25, no. 5 (2011): 1813-1817. doi: 10.1016/j.foodhyd.2011.02.007.

Gotthoffer, Nathan R. *Gelatin in Nutrition and Medicine*. (Grayslake IL: Grayslake Gelatin Company, 1945.) Kindle.

Hochstenbach-Waelen, A. et al. "Single-Protein Casein and Gelatin Diets Affect Energy Expenditure Similarly but Substrate Balance and Appetite Differently in Adults." *Journal of Nutrition* 139, no. 12 (2009): 2285–92. doi: 10.3945/jn.109.110403.

Knight, J. et al. "Hydroxyproline Ingestion and Urinary Oxalate and Glycolate Excretion." *Kidney International* 70, no. 11 (2006): 1929–1934. doi: 10.1038/sj.ki.5001906.

König, D. et al. "Specific Collagen Peptides Improve Bone Mineral Density and Bone Markers in Postmenopausal Women-A Randomized Controlled Study." *Nutrients* 10, no. 1 (2018). doi: 10.3390/nu10010097.

Kouguchi, T. et al. "Effects of a Chicken Collagen Hydrolysate on the Circulation System in Subjects with Mild Hypertension or High Normal Blood Pressure." *Bioscience, Biotechnology, and Biochemistry* 77, no. 4 (2013): 691–696. doi: 10.1271/bbb.120718.

Kumar, Suresh et al. "A Double-Blind, Placebo-Controlled, Randomized, Clinical Study on the Effectiveness of Collagen Peptide on Osteoarthritis." *Journal of the Science of Food and Agriculture* 95, no. 4 (2015): 702–707. doi: 10.1002/jsfa.6752.

Maeda, Kazuhisa. "Skin-Moisturizing Effect of Collagen Peptides Taken Orally." *Journal of Nutrition and Food Sciences* 8, no. 2 (2018): 682. doi: 10.4172/2155-9600.1000682.

Martin-Bautista, E. et al. "A Nutritional Intervention Study with Hydrolyzed Collagen in Pre-Pubertal Spanish Children: Influence on Bone Modeling Biomarkers." *Journal of Pediatric Endocrinology and Metabolism* 24, no. 3–4 (2011): 147–153. https://www.ncbi.nlm.nih.gov/pubmed/21648282.

Masterjohn, Christopher. "Vitamins for Fetal Development: Conception to Birth." The Weston A. Price Foundation for Wise Traditions in Food, Farming, and the Healing Arts. July 23, 2013. https://www.westonaprice.org/health-topics/childrens-health/vitamins-for-fetal-development-conception-to-birth

Melendez-Hevia, Enrique et al. "A Weak Link in Metabolism: The Metabolic Capacity for Glycine Biosynthesis Does Not Satisfy the Need for Collagen Synthesis." *Journal of Biosciences* 34, no. 6 (2009):853.

Moskowitz, R.W., "Role of Collagen Hydrolysate in Bone and Joint Disease." *Seminars in Arthritis and Rheumatism* 30, no. 2 (2000): 87–99. doi: 10.1053/sarh.2000.9622.

Nuttall, Frank, Mary Gannon, and Kelly Jordan, "The Metabolic Response to Ingestion of Proline with and without Glucose." *Metabolism* 53, no. 2 (2004): 241–246. doi: 10.1016/j.metabol.2003.09.013.

Proksch, E. et al. "Oral Supplementation of Specific Collagen Peptides Has Beneficial Effects on Human Skin Physiology: A Double-Blind, Placebo-Controlled Study." *Skin Pharmacology and Physiology* 27, no. 1 (2014): 47–55. doi: 10.1159/000351376

Saiga-Egusa, A. et al. "Antihypertensive Effects and Endothelial Progenitor Cell Activation by Intake of Chicken Collagen Hydolysate in Pre- and Mild-Hypertension." *Bioscience, Biotechnology, and Biochemistry* 73, no. 2 (2009): 422–424. doi: 10.1271/bbb.80189.

Scala, J., N. Hollies, and K. Sucher, "Effect of Daily Gelatin Ingestion on Human Scalp Hair." *Nutrition Reports International* 13, no. 6 (1976): 579–592. https://www.researchgate.net/publication/279548216_Effect_of_daily_gelatin_ingestion_on_human_scalp_hair.

Schoenfeld, Pam. "Vitamin D Supplementation: Panacea or Potential Problem?" The Weston A. Price Foundation for Wise Traditions in Food, Farming, and the Healing Arts. August 3, 2017. https://www.westonaprice.org/health-topics/abcs-of-nutrition/vitamin-d-supplementation-panacea-potential-problem

Schunck, M. et al. "Dietary Supplementation with Specific Collagen Peptides Has a Body Mass Index-Dependent Beneficial Effect on Cellulite Morphology." *Journal of Medicinal Food* 2015 18, no. 12 (2015):1340-1348. doi: 10.1089/jmf.2015.0022.

Sekhar, R.V. et al. "Deficient Synthesis of Glutathione Underlies Oxidative Stress in Aging and Can Be Corrected by Dietary Cysteine and Glycine Supplementation." *American Journal of Clinical Nutrition* 94, no. 3 (2011): 847–853. doi: 10.3945/ajcn.110.003483.

Seneff, Stephanie. "Glyphosate in Collagen." The Weston A. Price Foundation for Wise Traditions in Food, Farming, and the Healing Arts. February 1, 2017. https://www.westonaprice.org/health-topics/environmental-toxins/glyphosate-in-collagen.

Shigemura, Yasutaka et al. "Changes in Composition and Content of Food-Derived Peptide in Human Blood after Daily Ingestion of Collagen Hydrolysate for 4 Weeks." *Journal of the Science of Food and Agriculture* 98, no. 5 (2017): 1944–1950. doi: 10.1002/jsfa.8677.

Tyson, Terrence, "The Effect of Gelatin on Fragile Finger Nails." *Journal of Investigative Dermatology* 14, no. 5 (1950): 323–325. doi: 10.1038/jid.1950.41.

Veldhorst, M.A. et al. "A Breakfast with Alpha-Lactalbumin, Gelatin, or Gelatin + TRP Lowers Energy Intake at Lunch Compared with a Breakfast with Casein, Soy, Whey, or Whey-GMP." *Clinical Nutrition* 28, no. 2 (2009): 147–55. doi: 10.1016/j.clnu.2008.12.003.

Walrand, Stephane et al. "Consumption of a Functional Fermented Milk Containing Collagen Hydrolysate Improves the Concentration of Collagen-Specific Amino Acids in Plasma." *Journal of Agricultural and Food Chemistry* 56, no. 17 (2008): 7790–7795. doi: 10.1021/jf800691f.

Wheeler, M.D. et al. "Glycine: A New Anti-Inflammatory Immunonutrient." *Cellular and Molecular Life Sciences* 56, no. 9–10 (1999): 843–856. https://www.ncbi.nlm.nih.gov/pubmed/11212343.

Yamadera, Wataru et al. "Glycine Ingestion Improves Subjective Sleep Quality in Human Volunteers, Correlating with Polysomnographic Changes." *Sleep and Biological Rhythms* 5, no. 2 (2007): 126–131. doi: 10.1111/j.1479-8425.2007.00262.x.

Yamashina, S. et al. "Glycine as a Potent Anti-Angiogenic Nutrient for Tumor Growth." *Journal of Gastroenterology and Hepatology* 22, suppl. 1 (2007): S62–S64. doi: 10.1111/j.1440-1746.2006.04655.x.

Yazaki, Misato et al. "Oral Ingestion of Collagen Hydrolysate Leads to the Transportation of Highly Concentrated Gly-Pro-Hyp and Its Hydrolyzed Form of Pro-Hyp into the Bloodstream and Skin." *Journal of Agricultural and Food Chemistry* 65, no. 11 (2017): 2315-2322. doi: 10.1021/acs.jafc.6b05679.

Yoon, Hyun-sun et al. "Supplementing with Dietary Astaxanthin Combine with Collagen Hydrolysate Improves Facial Elasticity and Decreases Matrix Metalloproteinase-1 And-12 Expression: A Comparative Study with Placebo." *Journal of Medicinal Food* 17, no. 7 (2014), 10.1089/jmf.2013.3060.

Zdzieblik, Denise et al. "Collagen Peptide Supplementation in Combination with Resistance Training Improves Body Composition and Increases Muscle Strength in Elderly Sarcopenic Men: A Randomized Controlled Trial." *British Journal of Nutrition* 114, no. 8 (2015): 1237–1245. doi: 10.1017/S0007114515002810

Zhu, C.F. et al. "Treatment with Marine Collagen Peptides Modulates Glucose and Lipid Metabolism in Chinese Patients with Type 2 Diabetes Mellitus." *Applied Physiology, Nutrition, and Metabolism* 35, no. 6 (2010): 797–804. doi: 10.1139/H10-075.

Index

A1c level, 92, 93, 98

Acne, 46–47

Adrenaline, 101

Age spots, 45–46

Aging: 12, 15, 115; and bone loss, 58–59; and cognitive changes, 115; and collagen turnover, 25–26; and glutathione, 109; and glycine shortage, 28; and muscle loss, 69–70; and skin, 36–47

Allergic reactions: and collagen protein, 125; and histamines, 129

Aloe vera, 146

Amino acids, 5, 9–10; 102–13; chains, 10, 12. *See also specific amino acids*

Antioxidants, 108–11; 145–46

Appearance issues. *See* Beauty

Appetite, 87–89

Appetizer recipes, 163–68

Apps, for tracking protein intake, 27

Arginine, 29, 112–13

Arthritis, 14, 64–69; in dogs, 69

Articular cartilage, 65

Astaxanthin, 145–46

Author's experiences, 4–6, 151

Baked Falafel, 199

"Basement membrane," 12, 36

Beauty, and collagen, 33–56; acne, 46–47; age spots, 45–46; cellulite, 47–50; hair, 50, 54–56; moisturizing skin, 6, 40–43; nails, 5, 50–53, 55–56; wrinkles, 37–38, 43–45

Beef Bone Broth, 171–72

Beef Stew, 190–91

Berry Oatmeal Bake, 155

Beverages, with collagen, 138, 152

BioCell collagen, 39, 68, 70, 136

Biological value, 24

Biotin, 143–44

Blood brain barrier, 128

Blood-stopping agents, 18

Blood sugar levels, 92–101; low, 99–101

Blood vessels: and collagen, 11; and nitric oxide, 29, 80, 112

Bloody Mary Aspic with Shrimp, 164–65

Blueberry Collagen Smoothie, 217

Blueberry Protein Pancakes, 160

Bone broths, 19, 132–33; and digestive issues, 74–75; and headaches, 128–29; and leaky gut, 86; and pregnancy, 117, 119; recipes, 169–70, 171–72; store-bought alternative, 74, 133, 152; tips, 170

Bone broth powders, 152

Bone loss, 58–64; and aging, 58–59; and collagen protein,

59–64; and menopause, 58–59, 61–63, 80
Bone mineral density tests, 59
Breakfast recipes, 153–62
Brind, Joel, quoted, 104–105
Broths. *See* Bone broths

CAFOs (concentrated animal feeding operations), 134–35
Calcitonin, 61
Calcium: and bone loss, 58note, 59, 62–63; and nails, 52
Caldillo de congrio, 19
Calendula officinalis, 147
Cancer, and glycine, 102–105
Carbohydrates, 93
Cardiovascular disease, 78–82
Carnot, Paul, 18
Cartilage, 64–65
Celergen, 145
Cellulite, 47–50
Chemotherapy, and glycine, 105
Chicken broth. *See* Poultry Bone Broth
Chicken collagen, 67–69; and high blood pressure, 79–80
Chicken recipes, 173–74, 186–89
Chicken skin, 2–3
Chicken soup: and digestive issues, 77; and high blood pressure, 79; recipe, 173
Children, and collagen, 60, 121–23
Chokeberry, and cellulite, 49
Cholesterol, 81–82
Choline-stabilized orthosilicic acid, 144
Chondroblasts, 13
Chondrocytes, 64–65

Coconut Chickpea Curry, 201–202
Coconut Chocolate Chia "Pudding," 205–206
Coconut Collagen Coffee "Creamer," 161–62
Coconut Collagen "Cookies," 208–09
Coconut Pineapple Smoothie, 216
Coffee "Creamer," 161–62
Cognitive changes, and aging, 115
Collagen, 9–15; and aging, 115; and beauty, 33–56; and blood sugar, 92–101; body locations, 11; and digestive issues, 72–77, 85–89; dosage, 124–29, 137; FAQs, 130–39; historical use, 16–21; and mobility issues, 57–71; and modern-day diet, 22–32; and pregnancy, 116–19; side effects, 125, 128–29, 137, 139; storage, 138–39; terminology, 30, 31; topically applied, 6, 38–39; turnover, 25–26; types, 10–12, 133–34; at various ages, 114–23; word origin, 16
Collagen hydrolysate, 66–67, 69, 79–80, 82, 132–33
Collagen peptides, 31–32, 132–33; and digestive issues, 76–77; and heart issues, 78–82; and skin, 38–43
Collagen protein. *See* Collagen
Colloids. *See* Hydrophilic colloids
Conditionally essential amino acids, 10, 25, 96
Connective tissue diseases, 14–15
Contraindications, 137. *See also* Side effects

Conversion charts, 221
Cooking, with collagen, 138
Copper, 13, 143
Cream of Vegetable Soup, 177–78
Creole Cod, 195–96
Cross-linking, 12, 15
Cynatine HNS (supplement), 55–56
Cysteine, 110–12

Dermis, 35–36. *See also* Skin
Dessert recipes, 203–13
Detoxification, 108–10
Diabetes, 93–95, 97, 99
Digestive issues, and collagen, 18,
    72–77, 85–89
Dipeptides, 31, 32
Dogs, and collagen supplements,
    69
Donkey-hide gelatin (*ejiao*), 17,
    108
Dopamine methylation, 105–106
Dosage, of collagen, 124–29, 137
DPP-4, 95

Easy Chicken Soup, 173–74
Eggs, as biotin source, 143
Ehlers-Danlos syndrome, 14
Elastin, in skin, 35–36, 43–44,
    119, 120–21; in cartilage, 65;
    and pregnancy, 117, 119, 121
Epidermis, 35. *See also* Skin
Essential amino acids, 5, 9–10,
    24–25; and stress, 10. *See also*
    specific amino acids
Estrogen, 59. *See also* Menopause
Exercise, and muscles, 69–70

Facial creams, 6, 33, 38, 41
"Famine survival" mechanism, 84

FAQs, 130–39
Fetal growth, 117, 121
Fiber, 73
Fibroblasts, 13, 14, 37
Fingernails. *See* Nails
Fish collagen. *See* Marine collagen
    peptides
Fish recipes, 179–80, 195–98
Foods: raw, 72–73; traditional,
    19–20, 150–51, 152. *See also*
    specific foods
Fortibone (collagen peptide), 63,
    80
Fragmentation, of collagen, 37,
    41–42
Fruit Juice Gummies, 211
Fruits, and glutathione, 110
Fudge recipes, 207, 210

Gelatin, 5, 17–18; defined, 31;
    as hemostatic, 18; for nails, 51;
    types, 132–33
Gelatin foam, as hemostatic, 18
Ginger Chicken Curry, 186–87
Glucagon, 94, 99, 100
Glutamate, 110–11, 128–29
Glutathione, 28, 108–11
Glycine, 9–10, 12–13, 110–11,
    112, 117–18; and cancer,
    102–105; and collagen
    turnover, 25–26; deficiency,
    27–28; and detoxification,
    108–10; and digestive issues,
    76; in elastin, 120–21; and
    mental health, 105–106;
    and red meat, 96–99; and,
    sleep, 48, 106–108; storage,
    138–39
Glyphosate, 135–36

"Goldilocks Principle," 118
Gotu kola, 147; and cellulite, 49
Green Smoothie, 218
Guacamole, 163
Gummy recipes, 211–13
Gut dysbiosis, 18–19
Gut health, and collagen, 72–77

Hair, 50, 54–55; and keratin,
    54–55
Halal diet, 136
HbA1c. See A1c level
Headaches, 127–28
Headcheese, 19
Heart disease, 78–82
Hemostatics (blood stopping), and
    collagen, 18
Herbal Tea Gummies, 211
Herbs, and skin, 146–47
High blood pressure, 79–81
Histamine, 129
Homeostasis, and stress, 10
Honey-Banana Protein Pancakes,
    158–59
Hunger, and collagen, 87–89
Hyaline cartilage, 65
Hyaluronic acid, 144–45; and skin,
    38, 42
Hydrolysis, 31
Hydrolyzed collagen. See Collagen
    peptides
Hydrolyzed collagen protein, 17;
    from chicken cartilage, 67–69;
    and diabetes, 95
Hydrophilic colloids, 18, 73, 74,
    133
Hydroxylation, 13
Hydroxylysine, 30

Hydroxyproline, 9, 29, 32, 113,
    126; shortage, 30
Hypertension (high blood pressure),
    79–81
Hypodermis, 35, 36
Hypoglycemia (low blood sugar),
    99–101

Inflammation, 81–82, 86
Insomnia. See Sleep
Insulin, 94, 98–100; resistance, 99
Intestinal permeability. See Leaky gut
Iron, 96, 142
Italian Meatballs, 192–94
Italian Wedding Soup, 175–76

Jell-O, 5, 17
Joints, and collagen, 11. See also
    Bone loss

Keratin, 11, 35; and hair,
    50, 54–55; and nails, 50,
    55–56; and skin, 11, 35; as
    supplement, 55–56
Keratinocytes, 35
Ketogenic diets, 84, 87
Kidney stones, 126–27
Knox Gelatin, 5, 51, 134
KoAct (supplement), and bone loss,
    62
KollaGen II-xs, 68
Kosher diet, 136

Lacto/lacto-ovo diet, 136
Langerhans cells, 35
Lead, in bone broth, 133
Leaky brain, 128–29

Leaky gut, 75–76; and marine collagen peptides, 76–77; and metabolic distress, 85–86
Lemon Tahini Salad Dressing and Dip, 181
Lentil-Parsley Salad, 182–83
Liver, 82, 109, 110
Low blood sugar, 99–101
Lysine, 12–13, 24

Macronutrient ratios, and weight loss, 84
Magnesium, and bone loss, 59
Main dish recipes, 186–202
Manganese, and proline, 13
Marine collagen peptides, 134; and age spots, 45–46; and blood sugar levels, 94–95; and cancer, 103–104; and cholesterol, 81; and diabetes, 94–95; and digestive issues, 76; and leaky gut, 75–76; and learning/memory, 115; and skin, 41–42
Mashed Potatoes, 184
Matrix photoaging metalloproteinases, 37
Meat: recipes, 190–92; red, 95–99
Meat-free recipes, 199–202
Melanocytes, 35
Menopause: and bone loss, 58–59, 61–63, 80; and weight, 89–90. See also Aging
"Menopot" (belly fat), 89–90
Mental health, and glycine, 105–106
Metabolic distress, and leaky gut, 85–86

Metalloproteinases (enzymes), 37, 146
Methionine, 96–97, 105–106; and pregnancy, 118
Microfibrillar collagen, as hemostatic, 18
Minerals: and collagen production, 13–14; and collagen stiffness, 11; and undernutrition, 116–17. See also specific minerals
Mobility issues, and collagen, 57–71
Modern-day diet, and collagen, 22–32
Moisturizing skin, 6, 40–43
Muktuk, 19

N-acetylcysteine (NAC), 110
Nails, 5, 50–53; and keratin, 50–53; and nail polish, 52–53
Nitrates, 96
Nitric oxide, 29, 80
Nonessential amino acids, 9–10, 25. See also specific amino acids
Non-GMO products, 134–36

Omelet with Sweet Potato Twirls, 153–54
Osteoarthritis. See Arthritis
Osteoblasts, 13, 61
Osteopenia, 58, 62, 63, 80
Osteoporosis, 58–59, 61–63
Oxalates, and kidney stones, 126–27
Oxidants, 109
Oxtail soup, 19–20

Paleo Candy Sour Gummies, 212–13
Paleo Chocolate-Avocado Freezer Fudge, 207
Pancakes, 156–60
Papin, Denis, 20
Peptan F/P collagen, 40–42
Peptides, 6, 17, 31
Perreault, Leigh, 93
Pesticides, 135–36
Pho, 20
Photoaging, 34–35
Plant proteins, 24–25
Plants, and skin, 146–47
Pore size, 46
Pottenger, Francis Jr., 18, 74; quoted, 75
Poultry Bone Broth, 169–70; tips, 170
Poultry recipes, 173–74, 186–89
Prediabetes, 93, 94, 97, 99
Pregnancy, 116–19; and elastin, 117, 119, 121
Procollagen proteins, 12–14, 141, 142
Proline, 9–10, 12–13, 29, 76; 98, 112–13; sources, 29
Protein: intake, 23–24, 26; plant sources, 24–27; suggested intake, 26–27, 87, 93–28
Protein-Powered Coconut-Pecan "Fudge," 210
Protein turnover, 26
Pumpkin Protein Pancakes, 156–57
Pumpkin Seed Chocolate Collagen Protein Bars, 203–204

Raw food diets, 72–73
Recipes, 153–219

Red meat, 95–99
"Refried" Black Bean Dip, 167–68
Rheaume-Bleue, Kate, 141
Rheumatoid arthritis, 14
Roasted Vegetables, 185

Salad recipes, 179–83
Salmon Skin Salad, 179–80
Satiety, and collagen, 87–89
Scleroderma, 14
Scurvy, 14
Sebum, 145
Senff, Stephanie, 135–36
Serotonin, 107
Sesame-Glazed Chicken Wings, 188–89
Shrimp Cocktail Mold, 166
Side dish recipes, 179–85
Side effects, of collagen, 125, 128–29, 137, 139
Silicon, 144
Simple Pan-Seared Salmon, 197–98
Skin: 15, 34–47; and acne, 46–47; and age spots, 45–46; and aging, 15, 34–35, 36–47; anatomy, 33–36; and collagen, 11; and cellulite, 47–50; and dehydration, 38, 40–43; and keratin, 11, 35; moisturizing, 6, 40–43; redness, 46; and UV exposure, 34–35, 37; and weight loss, 90–91; and wrinkles, 15, 37–38, 43–45
Skin of animal, 2–3, 106
Sleep, 48, 106–108, 127–28
Smoothie recipes, 214–19
Snack recipes, 203–13
Soup recipes, 169–78

Standard American Diet (SAD), 72
Storage: of collagen/gelatin,
     138–39
Store-bought broths, 74, 133, 152
Strawberry Collagen Smoothie, 219
Stress: and amino acids, 10; and
     sleep, 106–107
Stretch marks, 119
Subcutaneous fat, 36
Sunblock, 38
Sweet Potato Twirls, 153–54

Tendons, and Type I collagen,
     10–11
Terminology, used in book, 30, 31
Traditional Chinese Medicine: and
     gelatin, 17; and insomnia, 108
Tripeptides, 30–31
Triple-stranded helix collagen, 10,
     12, 13, 17, 112–13
Tryptophan, 108, 124
Turkey broth. See Poultry Bone Broth
Turmeric, 108
Type I collagen, 10–11; and skin,
     36
Type II collagen, 10, 11
Type III collagen, 10, 11–12
Type IV collagen, 10, 12; and skin,
     36
Type XVII collagen, 54–55

Undenatured type II collagen (UC-II),
     66note, 68

UV exposure, 34–35, 37

Vegan diet, 29, 136
Vegetables, and glutathione, 110
Vegetarian diet, 26, 106, 136
Verisol, 43, 44–45, 49, 52, 136
Visceral fat, 36
Vitamin A, 13, 141–42
Vitamin C: and collagen, 13; 14;
     and scurvy, 14
Vitamin D, 141; and bone loss, 59
Vitamin K2 and the Calcium
     Paradox (book), 141
Vitamins, and collagen production,
     13–14; and undernutrition,
     116–17. See also specific
     vitamins
Voit, Carl, 20

Weight loss issues, 83–91; and
     hunger, 87–89; and leaky gut,
     85–86; management, 89–90;
     and micronutrient ratios, 84; and
     plateauing, 84; and skin, 90–91
Whey-Collagen Protein Smoothie,
     214–15
Whey protein, 88, 111; and
     aging, 115
Wrinkles, 15, 37–38, 43–45

Zinc, 141–42; and bone loss, 59;
     and hair, 56; and procollagen,
     13

Acknowledgments

Pam is grateful to her husband Adam for his loving and generous support throughout their journey, and to her three children, Jessica, Laura, and Alex, who (mostly) went along for the ride as she radically changed her family's diet for the better. She thanks everyone who encouraged her passion and love for learning. Finally, she is immensely grateful to her patients who, by trusting in her guidance, demonstrate daily the power of a nourishing diet.

About the Author

Pamela Schoenfeld is passionate about food and nutrition. She began cooking for her family at the age of 11, developing her own recipes with vegetables and fruits grown right in her family's own large backyard garden.

As an undergrad at the University of Maryland, she embraced the newest thinking on nutrition and health, which discouraged eating animal foods. Later in life, she rediscovered the documented benefits of eating nourishing animal foods. She returned to school to earn her master's degree and become a registered dietitian.

Pam has been in private practice for a decade and specializes in guiding women along the same path she followed, for both their own health and the health of their families. She rarely goes a day without collagen protein and encourages her patients to add a collagen protein to their own diets. Pam continues to measure her success by the health improvements she sees in her family, friends, and patients.

Visit Pam at www.thecollagendietplan.com, which features research updates, reviews on collagen supplements, recipes, and more.